STRONG ON
THE INSIDE

STRONG ON THE INSIDE

SURVIVING THE EVERYDAY CHALLENGES WHILE BATTLING BREAST CANCER FOR THE THIRD TIME

Marnita E. Kidd

To order additional copies of this book, contact:
Xlibris Corporation
1-888-795-4274
www.Xlibris.com
Orders@Xlibris.com
43306

Dedications to my loved ones:

I would like to dedicate this book to my family, especially those who are no longer here with us today.

This book is in memory of my loving mother Mrs. Joyce R. Kidd, her strong willed ways that I've inherited. My Grandmother Mrs. Martha Ellen Jennings, her silent wisdom, which I am learning to incorporate in my dealings with others and lastly my youngest aunt Irene C. Wimbush, you were like a big sister to me, I miss you with your classy ways of living life.

These ladies lived healthy lives, living it to the fullest, while walking that road dealing with Cancer in silence. Their unbelievable faith and relentless courage, and their love of life will live on in spirit forever. Rest in peace, I love and miss you all so much.

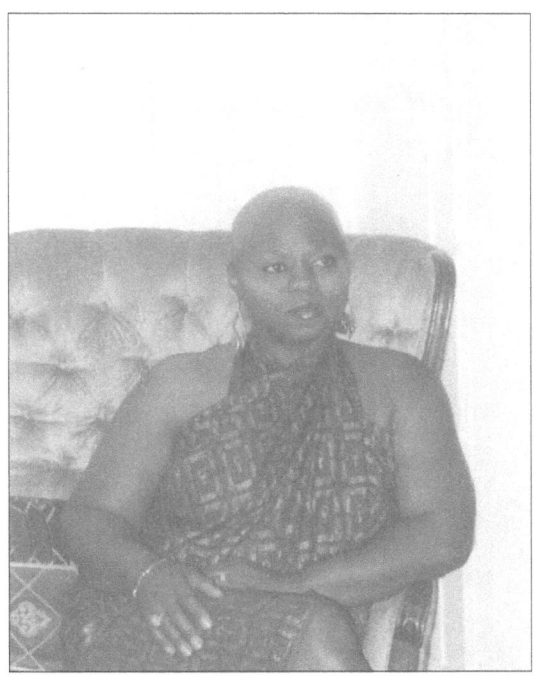

Marnita E. Kidd was born in Richmond Va. A three times survivor of Breast Cancer, retired Bursar from Temple University now living in West Chester, Pa., A mother of two daughters and grandmother of three. I am living with congestive heart failure, learning to smell the roses of life, taking one challenging day at a time.

A MOTHERS LOVE

I'm created to nurture,
I come in many structures
To give of my self is only natural,
So that you can be great in your own stature
You are a gift from above,
Truly as beautiful as a dove
When you finally leave the nest,
The pain will live on way deep inside my chest
As growth is important in this departure,
I pray joy, happiness, and love finds you in this adventure

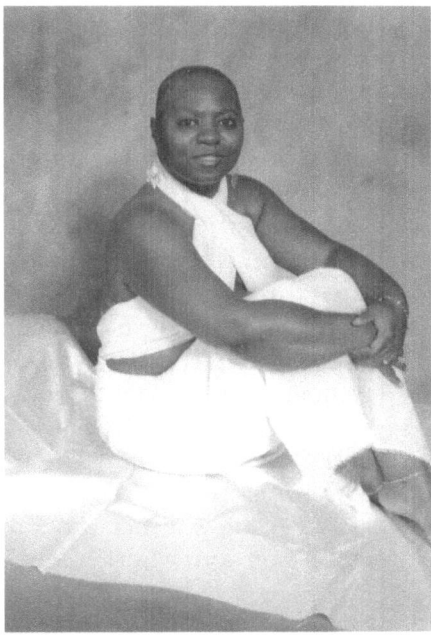

Strong on the Inside is about my experiences with breast cancer, not about my knowledge of breast cancer. Once realizing that I was in the dark and very afraid, concerning my own experiences with breast cancer, feeling alone in my illness inspired me to share as much as I could remember. Sharing with people who want to know, is one thing but sharing with the people who are unaware of the fact that they are affected even if it's not them stricken with the illness was the other reason, for telling the world of my struggles, while in my battles with breast cancer. I had an over whelming urge to try and express my own emotions, sharing the heartaches, sorrows, joys and blessings, during my battles with breast cancer.

I want you to know that I have never thought of myself as a writer. Completing this book I was difficult from the start just knowing that. Knowing I was about to share with the world things that are so personal to me. I know writing this book offers a great way to vent out to the world my ideas, thoughts; repressed feelings that harbor inside not only me but in my journals, secretly leaving me to feel disabled in more ways than one. My idea was to take some of my journals with my most secret thoughts, and feelings and share bits and pieces of them with you, as a form of letting go of some old clutter festering inside of me. Then I can make room to add newer, more positive memories to embrace, while learning to let go of my personal treasures at the same time.

That is what I am going to attempt to do in "Strong on the Inside". I am going to attempt to share some of my life's experiences. I've managed to overcome some hard times by having faith. Believing in God and not giving up in spite of the odds, trusting in the unknown of things, when I found it constantly difficult to believe and trust in myself.

I would like to start off telling you that I will began sharing my story with you as if, we were old friends trying to catch up on some past time, that we missed with one another. I will try to explain my experiences on, what it took for me to make it through my breast cancer battles, as I reflex back using my journals. Imagine us sitting in our comfortable chairs, on a bright sunny day. The room is a nice, but cozy size. The sun porch has a large window with soft, sheer, white curtains over looking a lake, with crackling sounds of water, bouncing off of the banks edges where broken pieces of tree limbs and barks that have fallen. The trees surrounding the lake are tall, offering a cool protective cover over the house, from the sun with its swaying leaves. The trees allow a nice quiet, but strong breeze to flow through the windows, in the room where we are sitting.

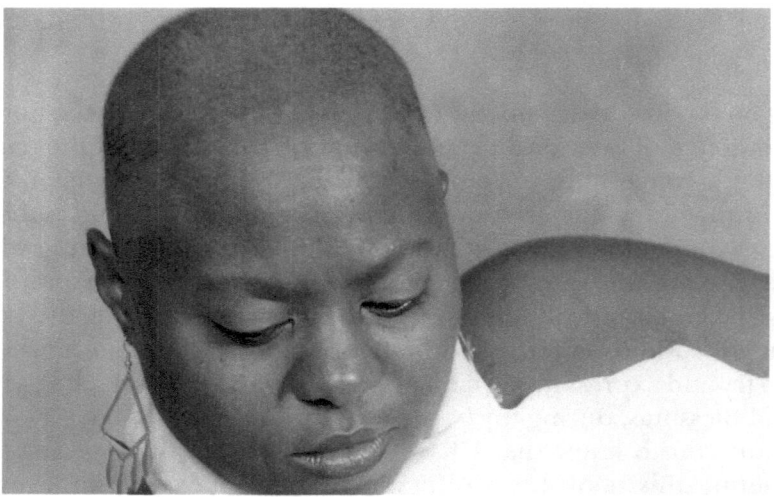

When you listen hard enough you can hear the tiny birds singing within the slightly chilly breeze blowing. The sounds of the crisp water from the lake out side filter in, offering a tranquil contribution to the soothing sounds, making a quiet symphony, or musical lullaby. These beautiful subliminal songs are playing just for us. We're comfortable in our blanketed covered, over sized, soft chairs. You and I are holding a warm cup of our favorite drinks. We're enjoying the soft wind blowing in, with the cool air to surround us.

I will share my opinions and a few personal photos, in order to give you a visual of who I am and what I looked like, while I speak of my battles with cancer, in hopes that you can embrace my story with a clear understanding.

You know the saying "it takes a village to raise a child?" Well I believe it takes a village of strong positive spirited people, to assist a cancer patient with care, while enduring their treatment plan, not just with their chemotherapy treatments, but all the way through to recovery, offering them on going care that is needed even if the person with cancer doesn't ask for it.

I'm from a small family. We're originally from Richmond Va.; my father is an only child, still living in Philadelphia, raised by his mother, who passed away long ago. I have no true memories of her, although I've always wished I knew her. I've never met any of my father's immediate family members, not that I can remember. I was raised with my mother's family. Being close to my grandparent's on my mother's side, which is all I have ever known. As far as family goes that is. My grandmother had five children. This consisted of my mother, her three sisters, and a brother. Now living are two of my mothers sisters, one here in Philadelphia and the other the other in Texas. My uncle has two homes. So, he lives between Philadelphia and North Carolina. I am the oldest out of four children. I have two sisters and a brother. One of my sister's and my brother reside in Rome Ga., and my youngest sister lives in West Oak Lane, in Philadelphia. That leaves my two daughters, both living together in the same home, in Ambler Pa.

I'm trying very hard to be open and honest with you by telling you that I am beginning to feel some great pressure from this third battle. I am not broken down mentally but physically it's extremely obvious to me, and to anyone who is close enough to know me, can see that these challenges are finally getting the best of me. You wouldn't know unless I actually decide to share with you, that I was feeling frustrated or unhealthy that particular day. You wouldn't know that my knees, fingers, or arms were causing me great pain, because no matter what I would still get out of bed, and try to have a normal day. I would try to complete my work around the house, as if nothing were wrong. It's something about me and staying in bed. I have become one of those people who can not stay in bed, unless it's a must. And I am not at that point in my life yet, thank God! So, I jump up in the morning as soon as I wake up, to start my day. I fear the moment when I must lay in bed, unable to get up, feeling helpless or heavily medicated, unable to physically respond to the people I love and care about, while my spirit is healthy and as strong as the day I was born. It has occurred to me that my body is much more fragile than ever, which is hard to accept. My body is a little more broken down from the repercussions of the recurring breast cancer also the daily use of so many therapeutic chemicals that were needed for the directly related heart condition. The other thing was the continuing surgeries for reconstruction of the breasts, and a hysterectomy which was prevention for uterus cancer. It's easy to understand why I would not feel as young as I normally felt, just knowing that.

It really has been years now with the recurring cancer battles. Taking the genetics test didn't help much, and I say that only because I worry even more now since I've had the gene test done. Actually, more than ever now I find that I can not help but to worry. I am constantly wondering when and where the cancer is going to hit me next. If I sit next to someone smoking a cigarette or walk into a room filled with smoke, the thoughts of "is cancer entering my lungs right at this very moment?" fill my mind. Other thoughts of "am I inhaling cancer into my body?" I'm always wondering how much time, will I have here with my loved ones, especially the children. People are always yelling at me, saying things like, don't claim it! I'm not claiming it but you know what you know, right? You feel what you feel. Afraid! I wonder if my grandchildren will remember me. I want the children in our family to have a lasting memory of me. There are times, when I wonder if anyone really cares about my, concerns and expectations. Why should they care? They have their own lives to contend with, so why should they stop everything for me. My mind frame or way of thinking is so intense now, after dealing with breast cancer. This is my life and because it's my life I am talking about, it makes overly passionate with the subject. I'm an empathetic person to begin with, the type of person who can honestly put herself into anther persons shoes. It's one of my personality traits. It's true! This time I am learning to be strict concerning my own happiness and wellbeing. Especially, with the things, I have always wanted to complete in life. I find myself wondering about questions such as how much time do I have left, because I am still wanting to do so much more with my life.

There are times when I feel I am watching the sand in a sandglass, running out of time, knowing I am not finished doing what I wanted to do in my life and there are times when everything is right with the world. As acceptance kicks in calming me for that moment, and the anxiety has eased off. There are times when I regret that I took that genetics test. Spiritually it continuously works on my soul knowing what I know now . . . Well, that's not all true. That's my fear talking believe me knowing is better! I know it is better to know if you are passing something like this gene on to your children. Also you can make preventive decisions to add years onto you life.

Please do not let fear keep you from taking the genetics test. Make sure you take the genetics test for yourself and your family's sake. How can I say I love my family and not leave information, on my life's medical history and experiences? I will offer my family as much written information on the reoccurring affects of the family's medical illness as I can, it will be the best gift ever. I love my little family. I am thinking about the generation to come, wanting and needing to leave them some useful information.

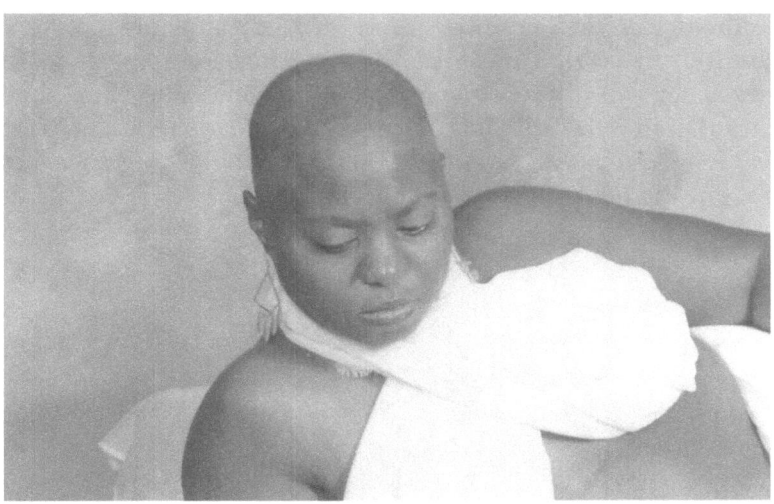

I love my two daughters so much, as well as my sisters and brother, my grandchildren, nieces and nephew, aunts and uncles. Therefore, I desperately wanted and needed to leave information for all of them, and other family members who need to have a clearer idea and understanding of what this challenge was like for me. I know there are a few people in my life who didn't take my cancer battles as serious as I believe they should have while I was in my fight. Their lack of presence simply showed me that, their concern level wasn't where I felt it should have been. So, I asked my oldest daughter out of curiosity, and some disappointment. Being a little hurt and wanting to know the reason for their actions or should I say lack of action, when it concerned me and my health issues pushed me to ask the question. I wanted to know where everyone was when I needed them. So, my oldest daughter explained it to me that they were "busy" with their own lives. I know she is telling me the truth but how busy are you for your own mother, sister, or niece? This crushed my heart immensely just hearing it. Believe it or not that is what she said to me, and with so much conviction behind it, I felt she was aggravated because I asked. I believe fear of the unknown can also make family members and close friends keep their distance. My friend and caregiver Sharrie actually had to bait my aunt who resides here in Chestnut Hill to come into the house to see me after my last surgery. My aunt wanted to bring me a basket of fruit, but she was so afraid to bring the basket, up to the bedroom where I was resting. Fear kept my aunt away. I really tried extra hard not to look as sick as I was feeling, knowing she was stopping over to see me. The last thing I wanted was to bring back hurtful feelings for her. Knowing our family's history with cancer is frightening for them. I know she has lost her mother and two sisters and now fearing my possible demise will never be good for her. As for my daughters, like most children they don't understand, until they are actually standing in my shoes. They will not understand until it's time. These are shoes I do not want them to ware. So, I just learn to save my breath and let God show them when it's time. I am not saying I want them to experience any of my hardship but life has its lessons for all of us.

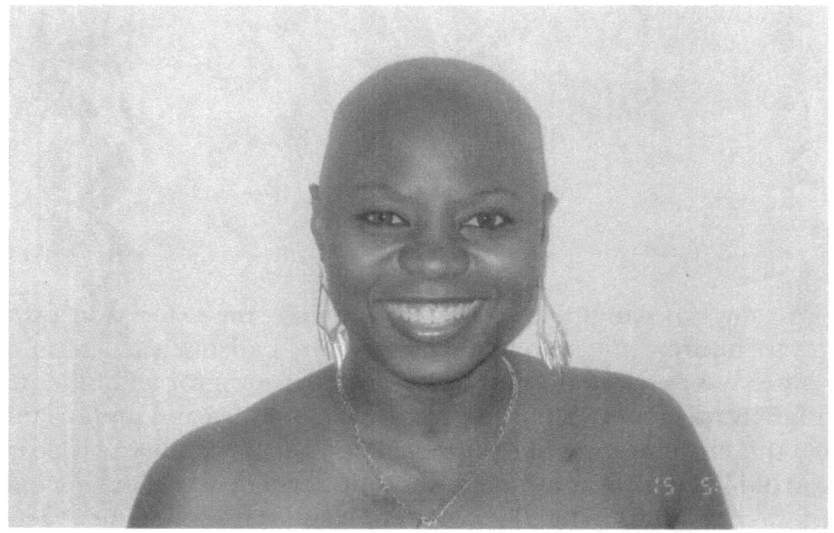

Bald headed in the bathroom.

People tend to people sit back and wait for bad news saying "call me when I need to come." That's after the person (which would have been me) passes away. That's not real nice to know, but again true. Then everyone would make plans to come make funeral plans, burry me and after the funeral have a party to celebrate my home going, moving on all in the same day. That's how it works in my family anyway. I would like to have my visitors come to see me, while I am fighting and alive! You know the saying "Don't bring me flowers when I'm gone"? I am a pretty normal person, so I think anyway. Others may say differently. But, I am as normal as they come and I have learned that I want my flowers now, while I can enjoy them. I also want my hugs, kisses, love and appreciation now!

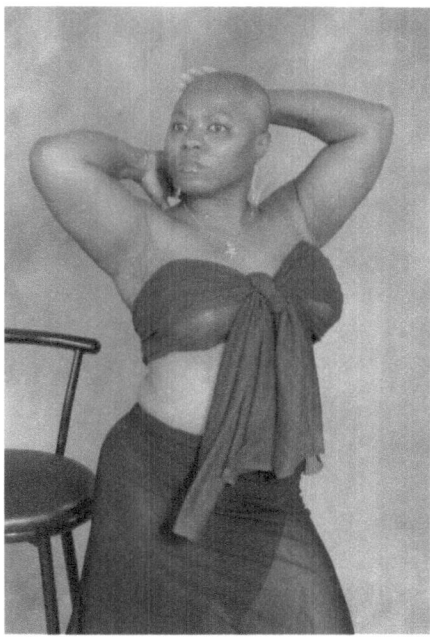

Gods work in progress

Forgive me but, your fear and waiting for the "person" to pass away from cancer is not an acceptable reason for any family member to stay away. The person dealing with cancer needs you, right then! They need a lot of encouragement and support and continued support. I do not feel I or anyone else in this battle should track anyone down, to mention the fact that I need some help. And really most of the time, all I needed was to have the presence, of my friends or family members. Having your loved ones around you offers more relief, than the medication prescribed.

To have my love ones around regularly would have, created an even more positive loving energy, offering the type of encouragement and support needed at the time. Assuring me that holding on and fighting through all the pain and sickness in order to recover, would be worth it all. Battling cancer is an agonizing recovery process, one that test you faith, in many ways. I began to see things that disappointment me greatly.

Not just in my own family but in people in general, neighbors, corporations, bill collectors, health insurances companies even medical office staff. Not everyone, so don't misunderstand me. People will surprise you from time to time. I've experienced others that conducted themselves in a way I felt I should have been handled throughout those unbearable times in my life. Watching them go out of their way all the way through my recovery was a great blessing. Also, learning when to move on and not stay in a bad situation, no matter how special or sacred. When I was made to feel uncomfortable or uneasy, fearing I was letting down my own family in my fight for life wasn't easy. I was the type of person who would always try to make the best out of a bad thing. Being a person who has made some really bad choices in her life time, I would know how to make the best of things. Some things are just out of our control. I wasn't happy, with the way I was left alone to feel fearful and secluded, alone in my struggles.

It is hard to be a passionate person in an extremely egotistical world. I realized how self-centered, inconsiderate, and superficial the world really is, particularly towards those who are less likely to keep up on their own, when I was wondering about my own future. People would see me, even hear me and still they turn away and continue acting as if they have no idea that I am existing with this illness. You would not have believed I was battling with a disabling, let alone life threatening illness if you were in my presence, unless I decided to tell you.

Knowing that cancer has threatened my family so many times would personally make me want to know everything there is to know about cancer. Not just by hearsay but first hand. Having compassion and love for the person would make me want to be closer to them if anything. Helping them in any way, would be my first line of action. Even if it is on a scale of a simple phone call to say "are you okay, alone, how are you today or has anyone been there to help you out?"

There were many times when I myself sat back wondering where my own family and good friends were. Not everyone let me make that clear, first! I would wonder if they even remembered that I was fighting for my life. Not to mention while I was secretly dealing with my own greatest fear, of losing my life. I was afraid, just like anyone else would be facing this illness. One night I had an idea looking at the old journals behind my dresser with dust covering them.

I looked through a few of my journals, coming to a decision. I was thinking it was not a good idea to hold on to a bunch of old journals. It wasn't going to do me any good keeping them. The journals were just sitting in different places of the house, collecting dust for someone to eventually come along to throw them away. The thought of that happening just upsets me even further. To think that my personal feelings, experiences and secret thoughts being thrown away by a bunch of none caring people as if I never existed motivated me to put the journals together to create a book.

The people who wake up finding that they, really need to know about the struggles that may accrue, during treatment and recovery with cancer, the ups and downs even if it's not them with the illness, may find my book somewhat informative, and then again it may not. This book has become very important to me as I reflected back on my experience with breast cancer. My experiences with cancer started with my own family members, close friends to my own fight dealing with this illness.

The response of others has become a big concern for me. I want people to understand what we are feeling and to know how they appear to us. I know that the need for clarification differs from person to person depending on the life support received. Some people have all the support in the world while others have to stand as strong as they can all on their own, as the world looks away. I'm concerned about those in their battle with cancer, who may feel alone and frustrated as I did for many years even with the little support.

For me, not knowing what was happening to me, and not feeling comfortable, enough to ask anyone who had to get through the battle was tough. If you are too busy or unavailable emotionally to reach out and help someone you love and say you care about, out of fear is another reason for this book. I've been affected by cancer in so many ways, making some turn away with, what I think are automatic thoughts of my dome, that intensified the fear inside me. Which is the last thing I needed at a time like this, we should look at fighting breast cancer or any cancer as just a different walk in this life time.

For example childbirth or divorce both very painful and hard to get through but you will survive the complications, given enough time. I believe in that saying "What doesn't kill you, can only make you stronger".

We are affected by these things in big ways because they give us a depth of understanding and knowledge that changes us forever. We are not meant to stay the same person throughout our lives anyway, growth in some direction is important. I believe having a positive perception when dealing with anything as great as our battles with caner is essential as well. I've always said no matter how things turned out I was going to be alright. What I meant was if in any case, if I did not survive my battle, spiritually I know deep inside of me that I had given all I could to the fight. Just like the serenity prayer, I hope you know it.

The Serenity Prayer:

> God grant me the Serenity to accept the things I cannot. Courage to change the things I can and Wisdom to know the difference, Living one day at a time, Enjoying one moment at a time, Accepting hardship as a pathway to peace. Taking as he did the sinful world as it is, not as I would have it, trusting that he will make all things right if I surrender to his will, that I will be reasonably happy in this life, and supremely happy forever in the next Amen.

This prayer kept me with an open and clear mind which helped me to weigh out the hard decisions leading down to the very way I would like to spend my days or accepting the way my day ended up when it didn't go the way I wanted. For example not just reading a good book but the entire comfort of a choice sofa or table in my favorite breakfast restaurant, where I know I wouldn't be disturbed, which, would leave me the freedom to be totally absorbed in whatever I was reading. Or to know that the pleasure of working in my yard, never feeling as if it was work but to know that planting this or that flower, bush or plant is a piece of me that will continue on as long as mother nature allows.

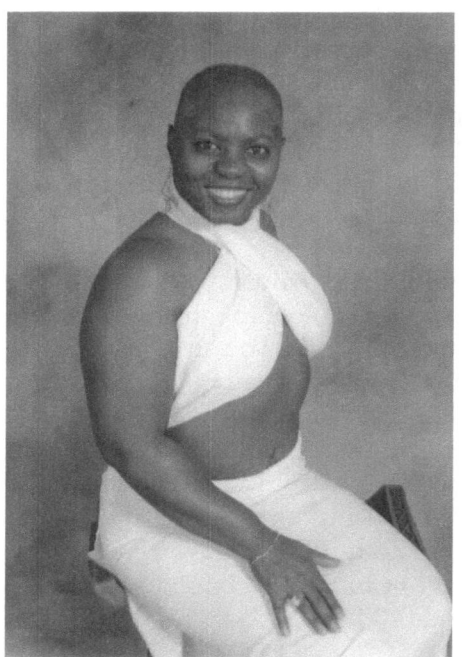 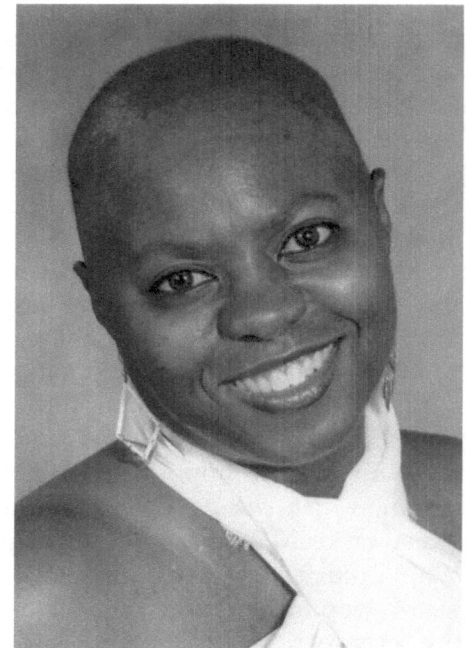

A Love triangle: My relationship between me, my medicine and a healthier balanced life.

Brightening my day when I felt I had no control over anything in my life. I didn't' care if my plant cost as little as two dollars, working to make it just as special as an expensive plant brought me joy. To marvel over that the two dollar plant was all I could manage in the first place, and see the plants beauty magnified with a little extra love and attention, proving it to be no different from the expensive plants made me even happier. Please, tap into your own hidden talents, as a diversion to what you are feeling inside to get through your treatment plan. It is also healthy to keep positive people around to lift our spirits emotionally to withstand all there is to endure with the treatment plan set up for recovery. It will seem like a long road a head, negative people will only bring you down further than you are, causing you to test your own will for life itself.

Don't feel bad to separate yourself from the negative people. It will become clear who they are, and even though they may have been a big part of your life you need to be surrounded by steadfast positive people during this time. What we do is take the news from the doctors saying "You have breast cancer" as an automatic death notice.

Which gave me an automatic option of letting go after a few battles, and looking at what I used to do on a day to day basis, like going to work and providing for my family or even the things I have enjoyed doing with close friends, knowing all of this was about to change in a big way. It became very discouraging to think that my life was changing. My usual way of hanging out with a group of friends, and associates having fun was going to change. Being aware of the germs that can seriously interfere with my recovery was life threatening information to be extremely conscious of.

I've had bitter emotions with people who just aren't sensitive enough, to be mindful of my feelings, especially while I was in treatment towards recovery. I need to remind you, when you're bonding with a cancer patient it is one thing to ask a person to relive their reoccurring near death experience, it's just a bit much for them to relive. So, if you can see the pain in their eyes when talking about something that was so hard in so many ways to overcome. You may want to withdraw from asking those, need to know questions? Let the person know that it is okay to stop, if they aren't up to talking about it. Please remember to be extremely empathetic in your approach with this person.

Fighting cancer really is a hard to get through time of life. There are days when waking up is frustrating, because the night was filled with extreme pain and agonizing discomfort. Here is a tip for you. Do yourself a big favor. Purchase a therapeutic neck pillow before your surgery. Because, for a month or two, maybe more you will not be able to lay flat on your back and the drainage tubes will keep you from sleeping even in the fetal position. So, basically you will be sleeping almost in the sitting position, arms propped up in order to not disturb those tubes. I would read my nights away or watch television until day break. Make up a wish list of things you would want or need throughout your recovery and stock up on your favorite books, and keep them close to your night stand. My girlfriend Sharrie bought my pillow for me, and to my surprise, it has helped me get through those long tough nights helping me to sleep after being discharge from the hospital and the seemly never ending painful surgery. I call my pillow "My Binky." I love that pillow it truly was and still is the best gift ever!

Getting up just to take early morning medicines has become a discouraging on going aggravation. It's not the act of taking the medicine everyday. No, it's trying to figure out what to eat every single day, before I take the medicine. I was told to take my medicine during the times of 8:00 a.m. then in the after noon and then again at 8:00 p.m. What is so frustrating for me is breakfast food. Breakfast food becomes boring, choosing what to eat every, single day. This always leaves me wishing for some new tasty breakfast foods to start my day off. I know that I can eat a sandwich or something from supper, but that would mess up those meals. You can only be so creative after a few years of the same, old breakfast foods. And that's not all! Here is the mental part of being up so early.

Now you're up, you've had the boring breakfast and it's still early, the day has started, the sun is shinning in bright and what do you do with yourself after that?

Normally I would get out and go to the YMCA and take a class or two. When there were no doctors appointments to go to or errands to run, but when there aren't any appointments and no classes for that day at the YMCA, I'm watching the rest of the world having a life, people going to work, picking up or dropping off children, children rushing back and forth to school, dogs being walked or people rushing to and from the markets with loads of food for their families, or making their way to the laundry mats. While I am in the house wondering if I can scrape up enough money to get my next prescription filled. And all the while I can hear them complaining all the way, having no idea of how blessed they really are, through my eyes anyway.

Here is another little tip for you because I didn't know and I'm happy to know this now. If you have only one health insurance carrier, a primary insurance and no secondary coverage, ask the office staff if their hospital offers financial assistance and if so get the telephone number and a name of a person you can call, and look into it. It beats not trying at all. I was approved for a Financial Assistance Card which helped with the payments left after my insurance paid the 80% leaving me with the 20%. Well, this card or letter helped me with my 20% of the remaining hospital bills. The hospital accepted whatever my insurance paid and wrote off the rest, because I qualified for the assistance. You can also complete a form at your neighborhood YMCA, and see if you qualify for financial assistance there as well, that way you can enjoy spending time recuperating in a heated pool or working towards some therapeutic exercise while you are healing.

This is a personal war with very few solders if any to rely on. There is you and the cancer. That's it! Well, besides your external medical team and the treatment plan that your doctor plans out for you, using his or her little book of grouped cases. If you have or know of a loved one who is stricken with this affliction or any affliction for that matter, you really want to know all you need to know about what they are personally challenged with on a day to day.

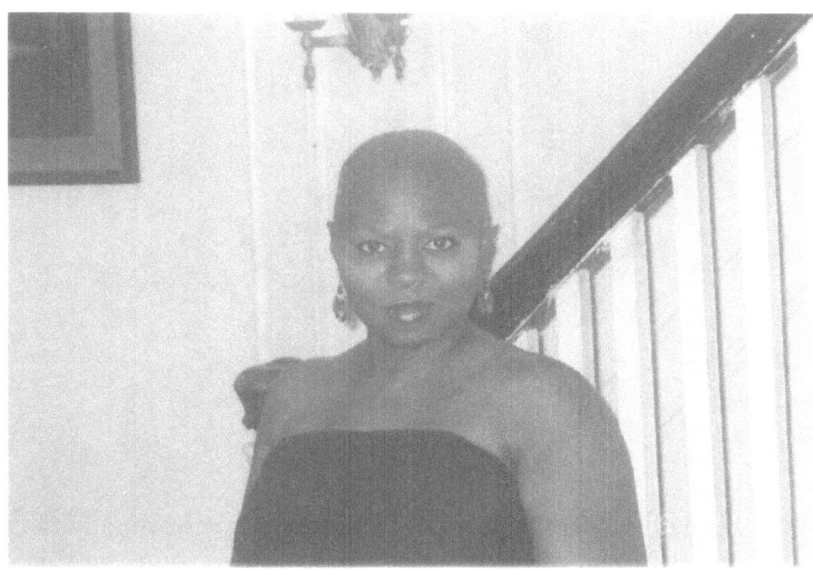

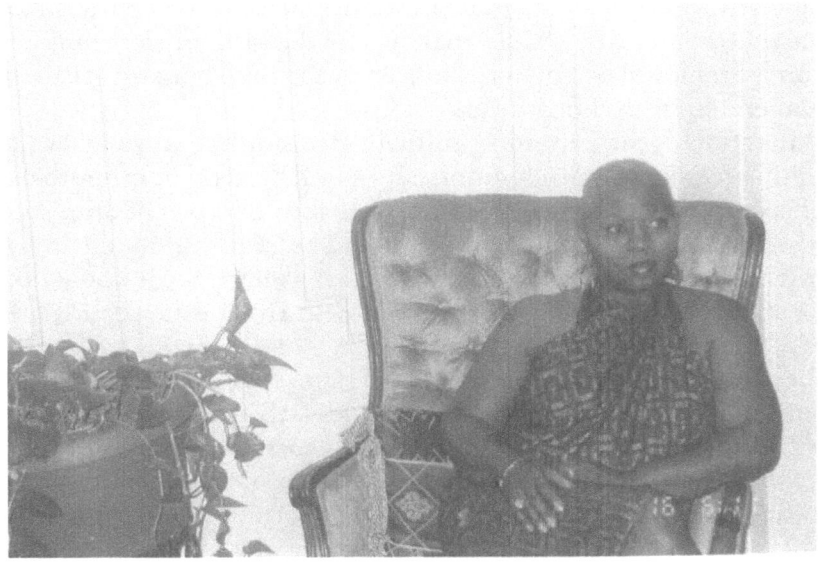

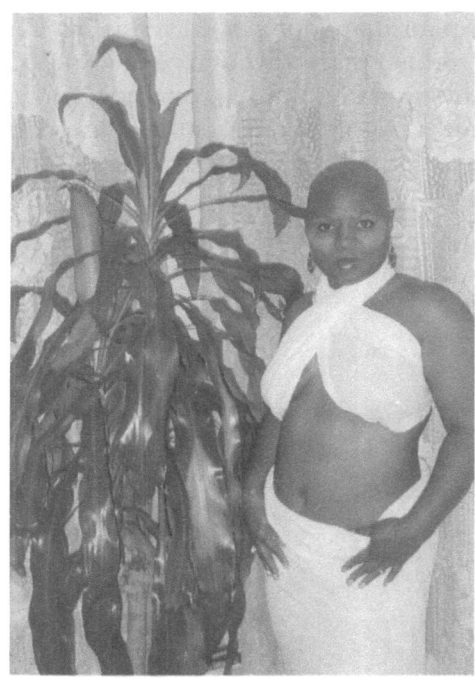

We really need to know all there is to know especially when it's a family member. This affliction can occur again to you or to someone very close to you. We pray that our afflictions aren't passed on to our children or grandchildren but it happens and there is nothing you can do except strongly advise them to take all preventive actions, or to not take oral contraceptives and to consider making the decision of choosing to have your breast removed or a hysterectomy knowing that there is a great chance you can end up with the same afflictions.

I know this is an extremely difficult decision for anyone but again something to take in consideration, and think hard on in order to extend you life, not just for yourself but for your love one or children's sake. I come from a proud family of don't ask and defiantly don't tell any of the family's business. My father calls me a squeaky wheel. So, it would take me to talk about my feelings concerning any disturbing issue particularly the issues of dealing with breast cancer.

The best way to do this is for all of us to start feeling comfortable enough to share our own experiences, with the idea that this can actually help others. That is the first step then offer gifts such as journals, pencils and pens, for note taking along their way through recovery. It's normal to feel over whelmed, frightened and in shock concerning the treatments used to fight cancer. If you are in doubt concerning anything, use the internet and Google whatever it is you want to know. Learn all that you can learn, and remember the experiences aren't all the same.

You see, I've had breast cancer three times. People always question me saying "three times" with a confused look on their faces? I've had a male associate make what he called a joke saying "but you only have two breasts?" I don't know if he simply wanted to make me laugh or if he was that clueless but he did not realized by the look on my face that his joke wasn't funny or appropriate. I was trying hard not to make either of us feel uncomfortable about what he said, but I really wasn't able to see the humor.

My battle with cancer caused me to be in constant turmoil fighting air if I had to, understanding that people just did not understand where I was in my fight with cancer while I was trying to deal with the everyday things. People just did not know how to deal with me and talking to them, was as if I were speaking a different language all together.

This reaction left me even more disappointed, if there was a way of being even more disappointed than I already was, leaving me to feel enormous amounts of depression. This type of reaction tells me that there is still a lot to learn, not just about cancer itself, but in the way we approach and enter act with a person fighting cancer or any disabling illness. The treatments used to fight cancer may cause many other side effects and health issues, which can make the person extremely sensitive and frustrated with the simplest things in their daily life of responsibilities. I've often wondered if choosing to fight to stay alive was the best choice. Knowing it is easier for people to be envious of me, seeing different people coming to taking out my trash or cutting the grass in my yard. Instead of them coming to find out why they see different people assisting me, often treating me with the same energy someone might treat a person with no common decency.

Seeing that people just do not have time and energy for your health needs or short comings breaks my heart. I am sure it differs from person to person depending on the type of person you were in their lives, may determines the type of support you'll receive when you need it. You have a judge and jury of family and friends collectively determining if you deserve support if any. While you are at a point where you are most venerable and in great need of them. But again in any case I could not take any stress, this was enough dealing with cancer again, at least if you decide to not show concern for the person fighting for their life, try to reach down in your heart and remember to be a little empathetic when you are in the company of this person.

During a sensitive time like this a person with cancer can make a sound choice to fight or not fight, secretly choosing life or even death. They just easily keep their secret from everyone, eventually diminishing with the details of their secret. Evident to those who care and realizing the cancer patient is no longer fighting or willing to hide the fact that they are terminally ill. If you feel like you will only cause them grief then by all means stay far away from them, because stress is the last thing they need. Send cards, fruit baskets notes or other gifts to say "you were on my mind". Well, you can get breast cancer three times because you can get cancer in the same breast twice and that meant an automatic mastectomy.

Which is what happened to me, I had to have a bi-lateral mastectomy and reconstructive surgery for both breasts, using my stomach to recreate new breasts. Now, Let us see if you can follow me, because I am feeling over whelmed about this, and it's getting to me real bad, at this very moment, and I want to explain to you what happened to me in my battle with breast cancer. I have a team of specialist dealing with my breast cancer and the congestive heart failure all located in the same hospital. This is great a smart move having a health team under the same roof!

Don't worry I'll explain the congestive heart failure to you because I will tell my story starting from the beginning. It's March, 2007 and I've just discovered another mass, lump or whatever between my brand new breasts. I'm still not sure what it is because it's under my chest bone, slightly to the right.

Now, you must know that I am freaking out? Well like I was saying before, the team of specialist from Abington Memorial Hospital won my trust many years ago, actually long before 1998, because I was seeing other medical physicians there long before my first breast cancer battle. Until now for the first time they've surprisingly made me question their intentions, with this new unidentifiable hardness. For the first time I felt that feeling of there is nothing else we can do for you feeling, when I ran to them with this unusual and very noticeable knot in my chest. The feeling was not enough to make me pick up and run way from my team to go to another hospital, but a strong concern with their action consumed me to aggression. You see they've ran all the tests like the CT scans, and PET scans ruling out breast cancer which showed nothing. The test came back negative! I'm relieved but I still can't help being on guard with my health.

Which, you may think that I should feel very happy receiving a negative test results. I was happy, for a minute, until I realized the lump was still there. Anxiety filled me to a point where I found it hard to swallow. I was sick to my stomach, just as if I had received a positive test result. I don't want to be a file sitting in a drawer waiting for someone to notice that there was or should have been further examination. Filing that result in a drawer and simply forget about it, was not working for me. I needed a follow up call, even if the test came back negative knowing my history. Plus it's on my body for goodness sakes and it's frightening to see it. I've also questioned my own insecure feelings thinking maybe I am over reacting, but to be honest with you, I'm not happy with the results and I'm not settling because there is something noticeably there and I want to know what this lump is, because again it is on my body, in my chest, causing me stress.

You just don't go to hell and back three times and not question everything. It's not easy for me to put trust into one set of test results, and you shouldn't either, especially when the abnormal lump is still there protruding out of your chest, and this one is between my new breasts.

So, I became very aggressive, making phone calls to the hospital, asking my doctors to tell me what the next step was going be concerning my newest issue. Because they've actually filed that negative test results away and moved on like it is nothing. Well, this nothing is my life we're talking about right now. Again I want you to know that this is a first for them. I took their actions very personal. As if the doctors placed me into a grave and walked away, without looking back.

Well, after my little unexpected visit to a few of my doctors in the hospital, without an appointment to express my concerns regarding their lack of concern, they decided to schedule an MRI, so they can look into the new lump a little more. I ended up with two scripts in the mail for an MRI and a telephone call from the hospital with the appointment time and date. (MRI): Magnetic Resonance Imaging machine—An MRI is a huge magnetic machine where they place you inside laying down, while you are on the table in a gown, it turns on and off again. You lay very still, holding your breath when asked to do so. I made an appointment to see my plastic surgeon so he can see if this lump is scar tissue that moved into the middle of my chest.

We should get paid to fight cancer, I mean it feels just like a job that nobody wants, and you work very hard at it!

I have some loving friends who offer, advice on healthy herbal ideas, insisting that I take a look into a new method to fight cancer and people you don't even know insist, almost demand that you listen to them and try their ideas for fighting cancer as an alternate cancer therapy. My experience held me close to the treatments ordered by my doctors only. Making decisions when you find out you have cancer is very confusing and extremely over whelming.

Practice using your intuition, question everything. Don't feel the need to sit there acting as if you understand, what your doctor is saying, slow them down and write down everything your doctors is saying or have someone go to your appointments with you so that they can take notes for you. If you don't understand you don't understand and it's okay. It's okay to say "I really don't understand". We all haven't gone to medical school. Medical terminology doesn't come second hand. To know and totally comprehend the terms your doctor is using to convey to you what the next few months of your life is going to entail, is not expected. Remember it is okay to say "I don't understand".

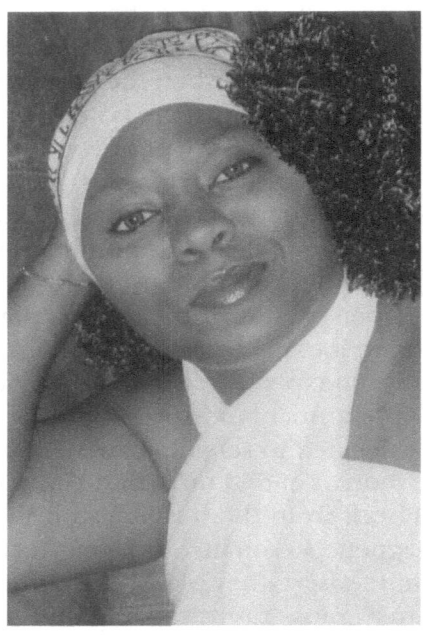

Also, I have had a few doctors that have actually told me not to worry, "Don't worry!" When a doctor tells you not to worry, go to another doctor right away! Please, I feel as if I've been through hell and they want me to not worry about hell! Well, this is something I can not comprehend and I never will. This lump may or may not be cancer but I would like to be sure, 100% sure, and I strongly feel if it is not cancer get it off of me so I don't have to worry about it any more. I have enough to worry about already.

When I met my girlfriend Linda, she shared with me that she had a lump. Every time we talked I questioned her about the lump. But her doctors continued to tell her that the lump wasn't anything to worry about, so why would she listen to me? A few years later, and now she finds out that, that same lump is the size of a cassette tape. She herself was diagnosed with cancer. With Linda, I had a feeling that we were going to be close friends; she has a warming smile and a spirit that is as gentile as a lamb. I ask her closest friends to encourage her, as I explain to them what is ahead of her, only because I know she is not the type of person who will fight. She really is a turn the cheek and walk away person. So, I try to make myself available to her in order to prepare her before her treatments. Advising her and letting her know what to expect when I can, so that she's shocked or surprised like I was. Not knowing what to expect was scary. I want to make sure she has a clear understanding on what to expect with every turn. Knowledge is power! There is another cliché from the cliché lady herself, that's me. I help her by filling in the gaps of communication, from doctor to patient. The truth is, at times it's unbelievable to see that the treatments for cancer aren't farther along. With all the studies, treatment plans and funds out there, there is still a lot to learn. Linda, Keep those boxing gloves on girl! Stay strong and know that you are loved, and you are not alone!

If you have any type of abnormalities in your breast, have the surgeon take it out! He can remove it and then test it! This is my life so until then we will figure out what this new lump is first. My health is first! Later I can focus on other things. It's not easy for me, being menopausal and knowing I have a gene that can allow "cancer" to sneak up on me at any time and any where. Never forget this, doctors are human and humans make mistakes! We don't know what Gods plans are for us, so keeping this in mind as a precaution just in case things didn't turn out the way I wanted them to turn out with this little abnormality, I have considered making preparations for the future. In case something happens to come up positive with cancer later on. I would like to have as much in order as I can, so that my two daughters are not burden with the awful details of funerals and other responsibilities while enduring the pain and loss of their mother.

So, March 9th, 2007, I made a telephone call to the Chelten Hills Cemetery to make affordable payment arrangements to finalize things. I am not claiming anything I just want to be prepared, for my daughter's sake. This is not negative thinking, it is realistic thinking. I understand having a CT scan and a PET scan confirming a negative finding for cancer is all I should need. This is what the Doctors tell me, but if you've experienced what I have been through, you would dig deeper also.

An ultrasound is small machine that uses high frequency sound waves, sends off in little pulse radar towards the breast. Gel is placed on the skin of the breast to make it slippery, then a small transducer is slid along the skin, sending the waves through it, when something gets in the way of the waves, they bounce back again. This is a great test but there are other tests that can be done as a second look at things, if you're not convinced.

PET scan: Position Emission Tomography—This test looks at the activity going on in the breast. PET scans look at how much and how fast glucose is being used by a tissue. I've read that cancer cells grow rapidly, so they use more glucose than normal tissues.

CT scans (Computed Tomography)—This equipment works by "visually cutting a part of the body into cross-sections slices.

Please do not be afraid to have any or all of them done. If you have the insurance get your doctor to do all of them. It is the difference between life, death and peace of mind. I just do not want time to pass only to find out that I wasn't aggressive enough this time around. Now, the beginning as I promised you. The first time I had to fight breast cancer. I was taking a shower when I found a lump in my left breast, this lump was closer to my arm pit really, this was in the month of May, 1998 when all of this started for me, and being fully aware of my body, knowing my family's history with cancer, it was important to educate myself on recognizing any unusual changes to my body.

Having an aggressive nature and being aware of my body helped me to notice when there was any changes or abnormalities. This also assists in early detection and a speedy successful recovery, from breast cancer. The next thing was to call my Gynecologist to see what she thought about the lump. She insisted that I come in to her office right away!

Without hesitation this is exactly what I did trying to hold my emotions in, willing myself to stand strong after I had discovered this unusual lump. Without any further delays she had me in her office the very next day, so that she could do the breast examination. Not looking too pleased my Gynecologist moved quickly, not only recommending the best Oncology Surgeon she knew in Abington Memorial Hospital, but she also made the appointment for me to be seen by him, the very next day!

I believe this is when I fell apart inside, crying in my doctor's office. Grabbing an entire box of tissues off the top of her desk, I cried and I cried. Her reaction was so serious about the lump making all of it too real. Before I knew it I was in the Surgical Oncologist office on the table receiving a large needle biopsy. He began to take some of the fluid by aspirating the fluid from the lump in my breast. The Surgeon numbed the breast as much as he could, but I could feel every puncture from the little needles. Wait, Did I tell you that I really do not like needles? Who likes needles, I know but I really don't like needles, and I've never in my life encountered a needle this large, not while I was awake anyway! The needles he used to numb my breast were normal, but the one he used to biopsy the mass was very large.

He continued inserting the smaller needles in order to numb the area. Then he placed the larger needle directly into the hard candy like coated Easter egg shaped lump deep inside my flesh, pulling out a large amount of a yellowish color fluid straight into the hub of the needle. I was ready to fight my way off of that table, because of the pain alone. I could see thirty years ago or so doing a biopsy this way but I just couldn't comprehend this to be a normal procedure. Not today!

I was already wondering if he was serious when he pulled out the large syringe. He sincerely apologized for causing me so much pain, and while he prepared the specimen to be sent to the lab. Seeing the color of the fluid he said he knew instantly, while holding the syringe filled fluid up to the light, that I had breast cancer. Just seeing the color of the fluid in the syringe, confirmed the suspicions of my Gynecologist, and again this was prior to submitting the biopsy specimen to the lab. I still had prayer. I prayed that the lab disagreed.

I prayed hard for all of them to be wrong. But intuition and good old fashion gut feelings told me they were correct. I just want to mention to you that this procedure was very painful to me and again out dated to me, so I felt but, keeping in mind very necessary. Again I must remind you that this is my experience with my battles. So, believe me as time goes on procedures change. But for then I held on tight to the edges of the bed, crying for this to be over and soon. I felt bad for the nurse because I had a strong grip on her hand, looking into her face told me she wished she could get her hand free from mine but, I wasn't letting her go!

The surgeon was very empathetic for causing me such pain. His face said I am so sorry, when he was finished getting the biopsy he needed. If I know now what I knew then I would have asked for (SDS) same day surgery to have the biopsy done while I was under anesthesia, sleeping comfortably. Of course, the test results came back positive. I remember falling to my knees crying hard again now in his office, when the surgeon called me in for the results. I had a close friend with me who lifted me up to my feet, while I cried even harder than I've ever cried before. I cried to the point where I was sick to my stomach, my eyes were burning red and sore, causing an instant headache that was out of this world. Hearing the results made me feel weak. Losing so many loved ones to cancer, I was simply frightened to death.

This lump never hurt or caused me any discomfort. It just appeared there without any pain, or signs that it was there. Nothing! When I was younger I remember my breast being so sore with my menstrual cycle. I would call my mother to ask her for advice. I eventually disregarded the pain blaming it on my menstrual cycle. Now, I wonder if that pain was a sign of something, warning me of breast problems that would come later in life. There are so many things in this world that are known to cause cancer, you just never know.

I tried to accept the diagnosis, getting ready for the worse. The next step was to have an Ultrasounds, Mammograms, CT Scans and all of the other laboratory testing requested by my Oncology Surgeon. Pre-admissions called to schedule the date and time along with instructions for me to follow the night before the surgery. There was so much to do and everything appeared to be going so fast. It was just the other day when I found the lump and now, what seems like two days later I am running around to save my life. Things looked different to me. It was as if God himself placed magnified glasses inside my mind. I began to notice the smallest most intricate aspects about every thing.

The surgeon preformed a Lumpectomy, removing the lump along with the infected lymph nodes. My Oncologist suggested a treatment plan using Chemotherapy (Adrianmycin and Cyclophosphamide) and Radiation. What I did not know at the time was that these chemotherapy treatments were the same ones my own mother used in her two battles, leaving her with congestive heart failure.

Using the internet when I couldn't sleep from being so worried about everything ahead of me, I would go into chat rooms as a way of communicating with other people using the same treatments. We could laugh and share information with one another, renaming the type of chemotherapy medication (Adrianmycin) "The red devil", because of the color alone. Adrianmycin had the color of cranberry juice. I couldn't even look at cranberry juice, let alone drink cranberry juice because of the color. The treatment took three to four hours to administer intravenously. Comfortably, I sat in a room in the hospital with other patients in reclining chairs, sleeping under the heated hospital blankets, watching our own personal television, reading, or whatever we like doing to pass the time away.

The nurses offered me a nice lunch and something to drink, with each treatment. I believe Abington Memorial Hospital is one of the best hospitals in Philadelphia, extremely personable. They are friendly, warm and they always seem to go out of their way to make you feel comfortable. I have had the nurses in Abington pop in to visit me, just before my surgery which offered additional encouragement and reassurance. I love that everyone knows me there, feeling comfortable with my team meant everything during my treatment plan, recovery and there after.

After a few Chemotherapy treatments, I figured out that I had a good four hours to get home before that day's treatment would begin to make me feel sick to my stomach. So, there were days when I was able to drive myself to the hospital for chemotherapy if everyone was too busy to take me. It became difficult to eat a real meal for a few days after a chemotherapy treatment. So, I would survive by eating Jell-o, pudding and lots of fluids, as long as the fluids were not red! I grew a hatred for anything as red as the fluid being pumped into my veins. The medication left a strong metallic taste in my mouth for several weeks. I couldn't help thinking I could forever smell the medicine, running through my body, as little seeped out of my body whenever I went to the bathroom. After a few treatments of chemotherapy my hair became brittle starting to thin and weaken, separating from my scalp but I was not able to cut or brush it off of my head.

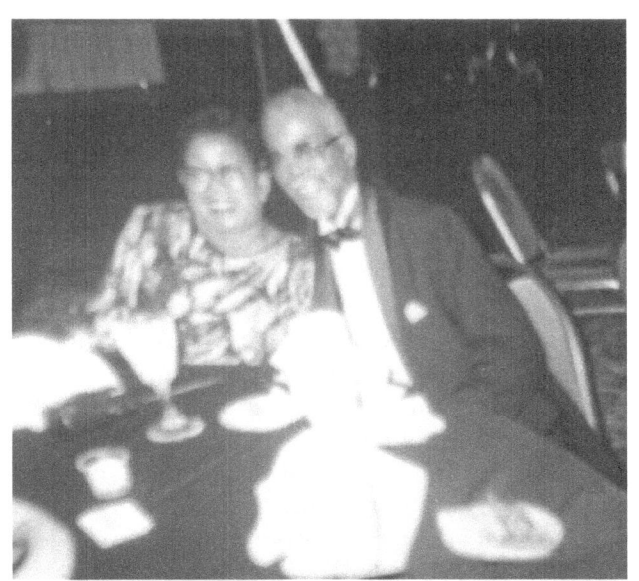

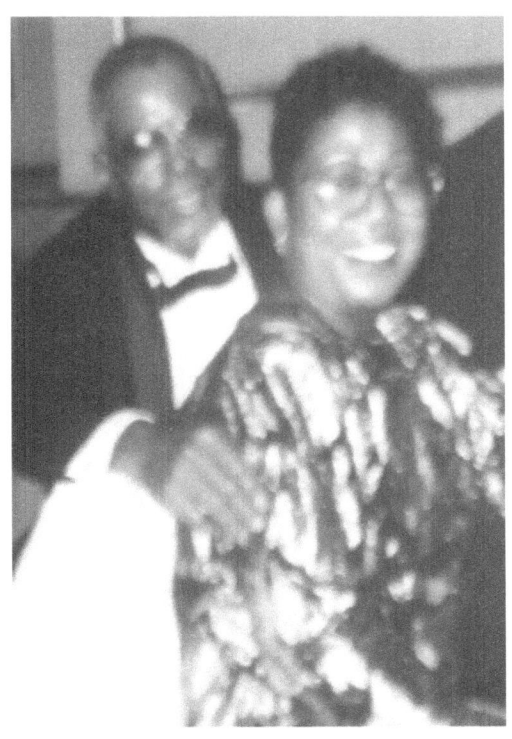

My mother and father's photos

Wanting to hold on to my hair became extremely important to me, at night I would tie my hair down with a scarf to keep the hair on my head for as long as I could. Until I decided to ask my sister if she could come and help me with my problem of brushing it out. So, I called her and she had no problem coming to help me. My sister, who lives in Rome Ga. Came to visit me on July1, 1998, we shared sister secrets while we sat quietly in my bedroom with the door closed. She sat on the edge of my bed, with me on the floor as she brushed all of my hair off of my head, placing it into plastic grocery bags.

Everyone else sat downstairs laughing and talking unaware of what we were doing. I remember her leaving me alone in the bedroom, when she finished the never ending job of brushing my hair. The sun started to go down as I sat right there unable to move in my darkening room. Touching my exposed baldness, feeling alone and very sad, listening to the laughter coming from the living room downstairs. I was still leaning against the side of the bed unable to move from the floor, waiting for my sister to return from taking the bags filed with my hair out to the trash.

My sister didn't know it but, she had my identity in those bags, or what I felt made up who I was inside. My hair was something I couldn't imagine not having. It's like makeup or clothes you feel naked without them. Exposed, transparent to the entire world, a world you were totally comfortable in, finally reaching your late thirties.

You know that age where you start saying you think you know yourself enough, maturing, believing you know what you like and dislike, without question? I was the type of person who didn't mind being alone. I could entertain myself, reading, sewing or exercising alone. I wouldn't mind taking in a movie or driving to meet up with friends alone, basically a simple yet confident person.

I became insecure in many ways. Well, I could hear the family questioning my sister as she went down the stairs to put the bags in the trash can outside. They wanted to know what she had in the bags. Still laughing, playing and having a nice time all the same. As usual, until she answered them in a slightly low but even tone, I could imagine her straight face and tight lips when she told them it was my hair. The entire house suddenly became quiet and for a long time too.

I wanted, wished I could have stayed in my room forever from that point on even though, I had a beautiful brand new wig that my youngest daughter Candice bought for me, but I was better at wrapping a scarf on my head and more uncomfortable wearing the wigs. Plus it was cooler to wear the scarf. Although, Candice made a very nice day out of picking up my first wig we shared a special mother daughter moment looking for the perfect wig. That was a sensitive day for me, but it was time to go pick one out. Candice and I looked in a few stores. That day I tried on one wig after another until we found the one we both agreed looked nice on me. Plus, the lady in the last wig store we visited was overly aggressive. She really didn't give me a chance to get all emotional over the reason I was looking for a wig, when I was feeling a little venerable. I was always natural wearing my own hair but wigs are popular these days and very much in style. Everyone wore them. She showed us a wig that you could get different styles out of and I loved it! That wig cost my daughter eighty dollars and it was worth it every penny, offering me an entirely new look. My new look was short and sassy.

The chemotherapy medication always made me feel like someone instantly turned up the heat in my body. I drew on my eye brows and made up my face, making myself look as normal as I could, and continued on fighting my fight trying to look strong. Let me explain the importance of looking strong, in my case.

Looking strong for me was something I needed to do, not only for myself but for my family. I am aware of their feelings knowing that we've lost so many member of our family to cancer that it's become frightening. So, keeping that in mind, I try harder to make them comfortable when seeing me. It a good way to lesson the fear in their hearts and it also lifts my spirit.

Now, on the other hand looking good can work against you, making people feel comfortable to the point of not calling to see if you need anything, like help around the house or a shoulder to cry on, visiting becomes limited and you're expected to act as if nothings wrong at all. This is my experience which has happened to me several times in my own battles. Feeling sick and weak and having no one volunteering to cut the grass, take out your trash on trash day, shampoo your hair when it's dirty, not even to see if you need something washed or a few things from the market.

People simply just go on with their lives without any type of empathy, when you decide to make people comfortable and chose not to show them your pain and suffering, be aware of the consequences in this decision. A few days later the only person I felt understood me went back to Georgia. My sister was gone, leaving me with the rest of my treatments, which came with blackening of my tongue and fingernails, and sores on my inner lips. I cried not wanting to have any more Chemotherapy. Finally, it was over! Happiness, doesn't describe the feeling I had once chemotherapy was over. I felt free! I remember smiling when I left the hospital floor feeling relieved it was finally over.

No more chemotherapy for me! I was tired of feeling sick. Radiation was the next step. What was I thinking when it was time to have my radiation treatments? I wanted a break from the Chemotherapy, but radiation was not the break I was looking for, it started off feeling like a nice break from that nasty Chemotherapy. So I thought.

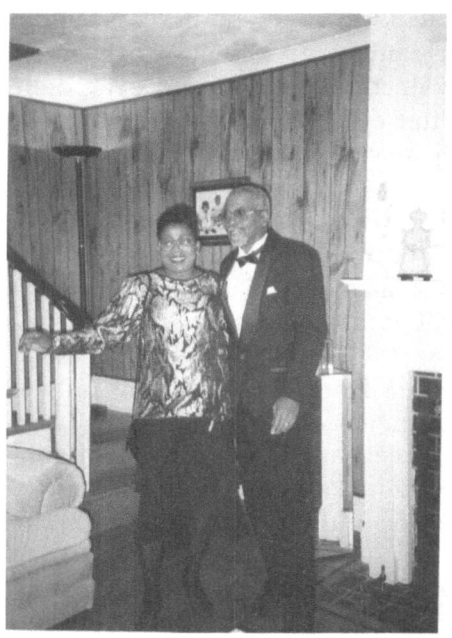 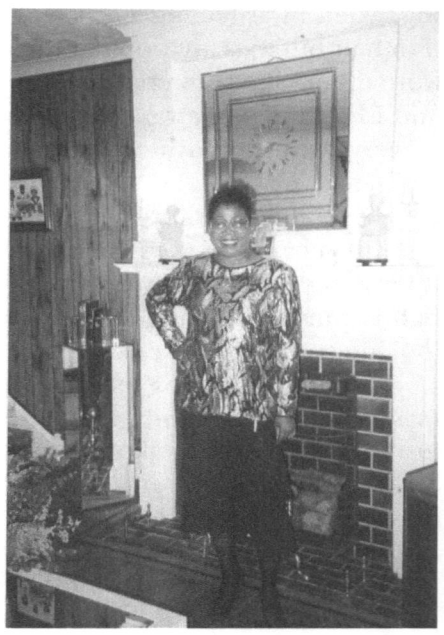

The radiation department permanently tattooed my chest, pin pointing the designated areas of treatment which was okay. Well, a few radiation treatments went by and I started to think this was going to be easy, but I was very wrong again. Nearing the end or half way through radiation therapy I started to realize a burning sensation inside my left breast which is where I was receiving the radiation treatments. When I mentioned this to my doctor he looked confused, and insisted on discontinuing the treatments he went on as planned. This upset me greatly. After telling the story to my Gynecologist, she called to tell him I would not be back to see him ever. She made another called to get me a new specialist for my radiations treatments, and I took a break so that my skin could have a chance to heal, because I was burning from the inside out! The radiations treatments were making my skin peal completely off of my breast exposing raw flesh. For example, do you know how an onion has thin layers? You have very thin layers of skin just like an onion and I couldn't believe I was seeing that the layers of skin on my breast was melting off of my body scaring me to death. I use an expensive topical anti-bacterial medication to soothe the discomfort of my breast. The name of the medicine is called Biafine. Biafine is expensive and was very messy when adding the cream to my burnt breast, every day. I needed the medicine and a lot of gauze just to put a bra on, especially on top of the extremely sensitive, exposed and painful areas of my breast. Believe me I cried a lot, at the same time I became accustomed to using a lot of gauze, and again forcing myself to look strong, completely normal or nicely put together. I found myself constantly wishing I had somebody close to me, to explain what was ahead. I didn't want any more surprises especially if they were painful surprises.

Carrying this illness made me feel alone just having the skin on my breast completely burn off from the radiation treatments, which was painful in itself. Not to mention the loss of hair and that includes eyebrows and all. Getting back to work was always on my mind. I had family responsibilities, long over due debts to deal with, and a house to run. Ready to return to work with only a few more radiation treatments to go, everything looked good, so I thought it anyway.

The second breast cancer battle was in May of 2001, three years later another lump appeared in my right breast this time. I could not believe what I was feeling, and yes, I found it while in the shower again. I felt like screaming "Is this possible?" All I could do was lean against the shower walls to keep from falling to my knees. I was trying to keep it all together, like always. The walls were closing in on me once again. Darkness actually filled the bathroom, making it hard to breathe. Wondering if this is the feeling before you pass out! Is this actually happening to me again I can't help saying over an over again.

Negative thoughts started to enter my mind. Negative ideas crept into my mind such as I'm going to die this time or I'm not going to live through this one. How do I tell my daughters? Will they be okay without me to call on, when they need their mom. Should I make plans in case I don't make it? Where should I start?

I should start a living will, but that would be too depressing, everything seems very important to me now, not wanting to claim that I have cancer again for the second time. I was already stressed trying to do everything pretty much on my own. I was still trying hard to catch up on all of my bills from the first breast cancer, repairs on the house and what about my job? I was just getting settled back into my job working at Temple University, and I wasn't sure if they would hold my position again, for the second time.

Forcing myself to go to work everyday until the test results came back, requesting that my physician call me at work because no mater what I wanted to know, right away. So, There I was at work waiting on the results of the needle biopsy, when the call came in from my doctor. We were all waiting for the call to come in, my supervisor and other employees, that were close to me. Praying, hoping, for the results to turn out negative.

When the phone rang, just hearing my doctor's voice made me choke up, as he began to explain that his assumptions were correct. The test came back from the lab and the results were positive, again!

I could not move, managing a soft simple response of "I understand", as he proceeded to inform me of the next step, which was to place a port into my chest above my left breast because my veins were flat, pretty much useless, due to the other chemotherapy treatments. I sat in my office hiding behind my computer on my desk, tears filling up in my eyes but, I did not cry.

One thing for sure, I could not sit there and continue working as if nothing was happening. So, for the time being, there I was frozen in my chair, with one of those smiles on my face that said "it's just my luck" to anyone looking at me, sitting in my office made of windows and glass, where everyone could see me. There was no where to hide. I know the look on my face told everyone what the results were, because I remember being frozen, staring at the computer as if I was attempting to complete my work, and my supervisor fusing about me, preparing to pack me up so that I could go home.

As a matter of fact she drove me home herself. She had one of the girls follow us with my own vehicle. Once we reached my house I walked straight through so I could sit on my deck in the shade of the tree with my hanging plants all about. They followed me as if they had visited my home many times before and we sat there on the back porch for a while, before they left me all alone. Eventually, they made their way out of the house returning to work. It took a minute before I could even speak. I just could not speak.

What could I say? Trying to be strong, knowing what was ahead of me. If I had to describe the emotion, I would say I wasn't in denial but in rejection. Yes! Rejection is more like it. I was rejecting the battle ahead of me, questioning my strength. Wanting to pretend every thing was perfect. I sat there inhaling life.

I sat there listening to the birds singing in the large park size tree in the back yard of my house that covered the yard, spilling over to the porch, the sound of the wind blowing through the trees relaxed me, and I watched the squirrels, jumping from limb to limb, playing without worry.

If history repeats itself, I was already aware of what the next move was and that was to make the next phone call to get things started, as my doctor instructed. This would make this entire process go so fast! So fast I wouldn't know what happened in the short time, while not even sure if I was making the best decisions, concerning my own life's existence. Most people get up in the morning and wonder what to wear to work finding that difficult. I get one chance to do the right thing concerning my health and future.

This is a recurring nightmare from three year ago. How do you prepare yourself for round two? I am fighting for my life again. Every where I go people can't help for telling me, how well I look. Even my Oncologist said to me once that he wished half of his patients looked as good as I do. I mastered the appearance of looking as if I had it all together especially when I wasn't really feeling well. He himself looked pleasantly surprised, and confused as he entered the examining room where I was waiting with a smile on my face.

Feeling good and looking good are two different things. Looking good helps people who know you have cancer deal with it better. When they come to visit you or when they see you in church, leaving out to go to the hospital or to the store to pick up things you need in the house. We have a wonderful coffee shop called "Cornbread and Coffee" I love sitting in the coffee shop reading from morning into the afternoon, no matter what the weather. I feel the need to make myself look as if I had it all together because I was in great turmoil, with everything. Things were spinning out of control in my world.

I was always strong and full of energy, being independent, challenging the traditions of life, and what was expected of me when it came down to the normal way of things. Being in control was always very important to me. It was nothing for me to be the head of my family, because we were growing up together. My daughters and I made our own rules up as we went along day by day. I was always ready to listen, help, and try to resolve the problems of my friends or family, even when I wasn't feeling all together myself.

When a situation came up, my thinking has always been to "stay calm, because I'm sure there is an answer to the problem and I'm sure we're not the first to have this problem." One evening while getting everything ready so that I can return to work, I was bringing up the last load of laundry from the basement, when I recognized that I was experiencing shortness of breath, when climbing the stairs, a simple task, which became physically impossible to do.

I was told I had Bronchitis and I was prescribed medication for Bronchitis, which was not helping at all. I was still finding it difficult to breath. Feeling tired for no reason at all, I was thinking that my body wasn't snapping back from the cancer treatment as fast as it should, also the cancer treatments left me feeling a lot more drained, this time. My chest continued feeling tight. I remember making it to the top of the stairs, this particular evening after washing clothes. I felt tired and out of breath walking down the hallway towards my bedroom. This can't be happening!

I remember placing the basket down on top of the bed and I sat next to it, but on the edge of my bed. What I could not recall was laying back. I was blessed to awaken after I had passed out in the sitting position, on my bed with my legs touching the floor! I realized then that I needed to go to the emergency room and right away! But, I did not want to go to any hospital. This is when I should have called the paramedics, but I was made to believe I had bronchitis, faithfully taking medication for bronchitis. Not wanting to call 911, and have an ambulance come, I made a choice and drove my self, in to the emergency room of the Abington Memorial hospital. I wanted to go to my own hospital, where everyone knew me.

So, I drove myself to Abington Memorial Hospital's emergency room, still thinking I had a bad case of Bronchitis. Arriving to an empty emergency room alone, which was amazing to me, I began to explain to the admission nurse that I was having trouble catching my breath.

They quickly placed me into a wheelchair, hooking me up to monitors that checked my pulse and heart rate. All while she took my history interring my information into the computer as quickly as she could. That was the fastest service I had ever encountered in my entire life time from an emergency room visit. I found it slightly amusing because I did not think I was sick enough for that much attention. They took blood several times, pricking my fingers, withdrawing blood from my arms, running test while I was on a gurney not even in a room. The emergency room staff confirmed and explained to me that my heart was enlarged and slowing down. On top of that the fluid in my lungs had built up which explained why I couldn't lay down without choking and coughing.

Everyday I took medication for bronchitis, thinking the coughing was normal. I was focused on one thing only and that was returning to work. It was explained to me, that my heart was slowing down to stop, not to be resuscitated. I was actually dyeing! Okay, now I am starting to feel an over whelming sensation of anxiety! I didn't even tell anyone except my slumbering dad that I was leaving out and he didn't know I was going to the hospital emergency room. I was experiencing a bad cold, right?

This was all going to be nothing I told myself, why bother everyone else. The idea of having paramedics come to the house at that time of night, waking my neighbors with all the noise, lights, wheeling me out and all of that drama . . . please!

The next thing I knew was, I had been admitted into the hospital not even aware that I was on the Intensive Care Unit, of Abington Memorial Hospital until I was being wheeled out of my ICU room for extended testing; the next day. While being wheeled out of my room in a wheelchair, I could see in the hallway of the hospital some serious medical equipment and of all the people in the world Pastor Gwendolyn Bond of St. Peter

Evangelist Church, my pastor running, in my direction asking for me. The joke is over! This is really serious! That is when everything really appeared to have stopped. It was as if I all of a sudden I was awakened from what was already feeling like a bad dream. Seeing my pastor was shocking to my system.

When you think of a Pastor running, through the hallways of a hospital, to come visit you and you didn't call, there is something serious to worry about. I was happy to see her but frightened all the same. I was later diagnosed with another deficiency called Congestive Heart Failure. I had fluid on my lungs, and my heart expanded to the point where it couldn't function properly, also there were clots found in my heart. Damaged from the chemotherapy treatments used to cure my breast cancer.

The hospital had to send a social worker into my room to explain to me, that I would not be going back to work and that she was filling out forms for my Social Security Disability!

I was being told I had the heart of an 80 year old person. I was in the hospital for twelve days with a 20% functional heart wondering how I was going to make it! Not being able to return to work, receiving letters in the mail from my employer stating that I was expected to return to work and when, which was 3 days from the day I walked into the hospitals emergency room. And they wouldn't be able to hold my position any longer. Talking about feeling overwhelmed. My mind just could not grasp on to any of this new information. The entire situation was just too much for me to handle. The second battle with breast cancer, no job and congestive heart failure, only God can hold me together now.

Social worker or no social worker I wanted no needed to return to work! I was trying to be strong again. I was fighting everything and everyone who was telling me I would not return to work. This could not be happening to me!

I know that Doctors have their reasons for telling you just enough information and not all, unless you know the questions to ask, but I believe this discovery was pertinent information that should have been brought to my attention from my Oncologist before the treatments began, knowing there is a chance of Congestive Heart Failure as a recurring side affect that occurs in a moderate percentage of people with a particular chemotherapy treatment, should have been explained. Not after the damage has been done, "saying this medication has been known to cause CHF".

Doctors should inform their patients that the likelihood of these cancer treatments may show side affects such as congestive heart failure. Breast cancer is no stranger to my family. The family members that experienced cancer have passed on. They did not believe in talking about "cancer", they tried hard to keep cancer quiet. Cancer was kept a secret, until they could not hide it anymore. Cancer has taken them away from the family, removing them out of our lives. I am different, my father calls me a squeaky wheal, because I need to talk, and express and share, what I know. No more secrets! No more being in the dark, secretly whispering to one another not having the full information. That's over!

I believe we should talk about cancer. Leave notes, journals and photos expressing the harsh reality of the nature of this beast. Now, I need a plan and my plan is to try harder to focus on the true importance of life. I need to use all of my energy to focus on myself. Learning to stay positive, taking note to what is important and what is not. Restricting myself to resolving my own problems first has become a challenge for me these days, because I am a naturally a caregiver. It is hard but I am still learning to say no, I can't or I don't have it. I had to exercise more often than before, working on better eating habits and work to create a real tranquil living space.

I needed to push away from anything or anyone holding on to negative energy. Being unaware, and not having any guidance from my mother with this issue. My mother who won her battle twice with breast cancer, ending up with Congestive Heart Failure herself, unable to stop working because she was the only bread winner of our family, she held together our home and four children as best she could, when she passed away with an aneurisms. My mom was attending our church, for a meeting one evening. My brother-in-law who is a doctor was with her at this meeting, when she passed away. He called me to say "Things don't so look good." My heart started to pump fast, my mind questioned what he meant. Disbelief locked in disregarding the words he spoke to me over the telephone. All ready calculating in my head the time it would take to get, where they were. I jumped into my car and headed over to the church. I was too late the paramedics, were closing the doors on the ambulance with my mother inside.

I could see a glimpse of her as they finished closing the back doors, of the ambulance to drive away. I never spoke to my mom again. I was unaware of anything else I didn't even realize that my father was sitting in his car, parked in front of mine, not moving at all, just sitting there in the drivers seat, with his head facing down. He was parked behind the ambulance, not moving, in total shock as I was. In disbelief, seeing his wife was no longer with him. You never know when your time is going to be up, and you'll never see that loved one again. We all followed the ambulance to the hospital to discover she had passed away. When all of the testing was done and everyone went back to the house, I just sat there in the hospital next to my mother in the hospital bed, just sitting there for hours. Until I could move and then I just walked out!

Leaving her and no information completed for the hospital staff, I walked right out. I was in shock, not ready to move on from that point. My mind went blank. I had no idea what to do next. This is unbelievable! Who says "One night my mother went to church and never came home"? This is a painful but true story. I've recently learned from my father, that my mother and I share the same afflictions, and at the same ages, which makes me wonder, what's next for me. Will I have a stroke if I don't learn to relax and settle down keeping stress and negativity at a bay? It is something to think about.

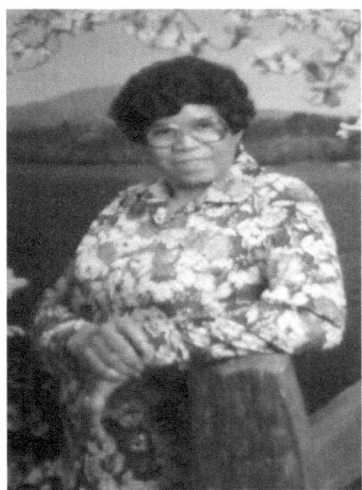 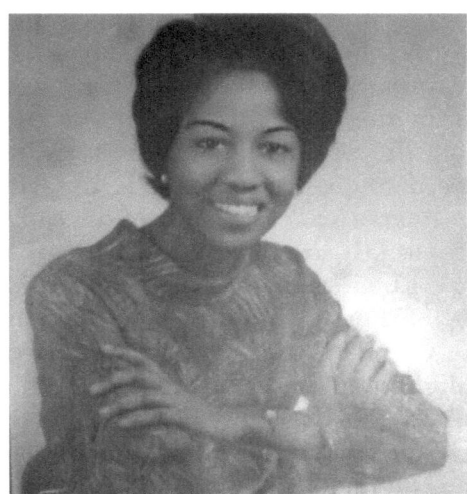

My Grandmother Margaret Jennings and Aunt Irene Wimbush

My youngest aunt (my mother's youngest sister) lost her battle with breast cancer at an early age. She was in her early forties, a model looking young woman, working for Eastern Airlines living a great single life, always looking beautiful and driving the classiest sports cars, traveling when and wherever she wanted, at times taking us with her when she could. I really admired her life, and I wanted to enjoy life the way she did. She was a very regal, a high energy spirited person. People treated her like a queen. She had her own way of making things happen. Demanding the best wherever she went, receiving the respect she deserved. She convinced me to get my drivers license, by offering to buy my first car. She made her promise good and I was a very happy girl. She was someone, I could look up too. This was my aunt Irene, the closest family member to me, she was much more than that she was just like my own big sister.

My grandmother who suffered with pancreas cancer, departed suddenly once finding out her diagnosis. I knew she had surgery on her stomach but, I didn't know it was cancer. I remember her going to the hospital and then coming home, nothing was mentioned to "us" the children about it. I watched her take medicine regularly, to try and ease her upset stomach problems. And then one day the family took her to the hospital, saying she'll be back and everything will be okay. Saying "she was just going to the hospital to get checked." My grandmother never returned home. My grandfather lived a few more years, and then he also passed away.

Now they are all gone leaving me alone and in the dark about the changes and reactions my body will experience from the much needed treatments and recovery. These treatments as harsh as it may seem, are by the book procedures that caused me to mentally feel secluded from the world I knew. When my life took a turn for the worse, I was not mentally prepared for it, but when you think of life's changes and your experiences, are any of us ready for it? I believe things happen for a reason. If you believe our lives are already planed out for us, which is what I believe, having my children when I did as a teenager was simply, one of those things in my life that was meant to be. Raising two children was very hard for me as a single parent, but my oldest daughter Tyesha enlightened me by saying that I made raising children look like a lot of fun. As a teenager I really wasn't ready to start a family and who is ready? But we (my daughters and my self) made the best out of life, together. I was eighteen with two children, trying my best to do what I could with what I had. Once we lived in a one bedroom apartment a duplex in West Oak Lane in Philadelphia. My daughters were so small, when I asked about that apartment they didn't even realize that the apartment was a one bedroom. They were happy and that's all that mattered to me. They slept in the bedroom and I had the sofa. Everyday after working in the medical center I was sleeping on a sofa. On those weekends, when they went to visit their father, I would get the only bed in the apartment and stretch out. It was ruff, I'll admit. Children grow up so fast, and that's what they did. They grew up so fast and moved on leaving me with the unexpected empty nest syndrome. A syndrome that's like no other, Instead of enjoying life because things could now be just about me, life only became harder. I ended up with my breast cancer battles and the affects it leaves you with in the end. I ended up without a job, going from church to church looking for free food handouts in all kinds of weather. Lifting heavy bags when I knew my doctors said not to lift over five pounds. I was determined and desperate to be independent. So I pushed on doing what I had to do. Always grateful for the small things, but feeling torn because

I know the can goods are filled with sodium, and preservatives the rice, potatoes, yams and vegetables, were not so great looking and were over the amount of starch for a healthy intake. The close to out dated cereals and pasta was better than nothing. And once a week I would run to any church giving out handouts, like bread, all types of bread, waffles, pita, wheat, and raisin bread. If you know how to cook you can make hefty meals out of these handouts.

Right now, I don't worry about what I am going to eat or where I am going to sleep, but I still struggle with the fact that I am unable to care for myself properly without help. Being dependant hurts me, deeply. I find it difficult at times because I've finished raising children, and I've retired and when I tell myself I need or want something, something small or simple and can't afford it, I break down. Buying from a second hand store was no problem either. But when you can't afford to shop in a Goodwill store, the dollar store or the thrift stores, you can become depressed.

I remember shopping with one of my closest girlfriends. Keeping a promise I made to take her out so that she could shop for her birthday. First seeing that she wanted to go into Talbert's, a store I could and hadn't ever shopped in was the start of some enormous anxiety. Going in and looking at the prices on the things I liked and wished for overwhelmed me with great discomfort. When she asked me to help her pick out things and she wanted to know if I thought they looked nice on her pushed me over the edge. Because, at that point I realized that I was, what I called "poor". I've been begging for food all week long and now I was standing in an expensive store with one buck in my pocket, holding back tears of depression that was really brought on by the onset of my recurring illnesses. I was experiencing "my bottom." After becoming disabled in 2001, my life changed, and not for the better. I realized to buy a new bra or new shoes would seriously take away from a greater need later on. And if you know me shoes are my weakness. I was just in love with buying shoes and boots. I had not graduated into pocketbooks yet, thank God! But now standing in Talbert's looking at price tags and aching deep inside, trying not to show any of it because I didn't want my girlfriend to know and I didn't want to spoil her day. But all the time I just wanted desperately to go home. I wanted to throw a tantrum and run out of there. But that wasn't that type of person I was, me I wouldn't let on to my pain, she asked if we could go to a small coffee shop not far from where we were. While I looked on as the clerk rang up the total of her purchases, feeling as if I was so close to passing out in there store. Of course I said sure, knowing I couldn't afford to get anything. But we sat there as I managed to get a cup of tea. While she sat happily eating something and drinking a special made tea, I secretly sulked because I didn't know how to say to her or out loud, what I was feeling. I've felt like this other times, especially on holidays and loved ones birthdays. I understand why I can't do for myself or others I care for, it's just so frustrating and very hard to accept, even today. I said all of that to say this, I was never use to having a lot of money or an abundance of new things but I've never felt this dependant.

Now, when I think back on raising my children, it was extremely for filling and so much fun for me. I realized today having my children when I did was the right choice. Most of all one of the best choices I have ever made in my entire life! Things would have been very different if I had waited to start a family. Having children completed my life. Holidays were upsetting for years, because I would always go to work, needing the extra money for my children. So, I would send them to their dads or my mother's house, missing out on seeing the joy on their faces Christmas morning. You know kids should wake up extra early, run down stairs to see what was under the Christmas tree. Not, wait all day until I came home, I would sacrifice spending that time with them. Our time was when I returned from work in the evening. When the holiday events and everything appeared to be over and they've visited their dad and other grandparents, we would head home. Thinking the day was over holding their collection of gifts. I would open up the door to our home with our Christmas tree filled with toys and other things. The look on their faces made the sacrifices more than worth it. They jumped and ran and screamed and danced their little bodies around looking so funny. For me that was the joy. It made up for missing out on all the other holiday stuff.

Today, thinking back, I don't think I would have had the energy to get through the three breast cancers, and related congestive heart failure, hysterectomy, and Menopause, while raising my two children as a single parent. Menopause! Why? It's not right! Don't I have enough to go through? My Gynecologic Oncologist explained to me that a normal healthy female can fight off a virus such as the H.P.V. virus. I had fibroids and cysts on my ovaries, which drew a concern to my Oncologist.

My body's immune system had weakened with all of the cancer treatments. Therefore, with my family history a Hysterectomy was needed, and right away!

Although, I was in the beginning process of healing from having a Bilateral Mastectomy and the Trams Flap Surgery, where one part of the surgery is a neat bikini cut stretching from one side of your stomach to the other. The Oncology surgeon preformed the mastectomy, removing the old breast and then the plastic surgeon takes over using the stomach muscles along with fatty tissue in order to create new breast once the mastectomy was completed.

I woke up with new size "c" cup breasts and a nice tummy tuck, coming to after the surgery was difficult because my mind couldn't understand the pain my body was experiencing. I had drainage tubes coming out of my stomach and from the sides of my breasts. On top of it I initially had my family and friends standing all around me, admiring my new youthful body. But the pain wouldn't allow me to be any thing close to happy, nice, appreciative, grateful nor hospitable, or anything like that.

Not being the sociable person I used to be, I found myself wanting and needing to be alone with my pain medication, in order to begin to comprehend why the pain was so great! Still under the influence of the anesthesia medication, and not really in my right mind, my family said I put everyone out of the recovery room, following my surgery. I couldn't share in the rejoicing of my new body as they were doing. The pain was unbearable to say the least.

It's now the beginning of the year 2006 and I am 44 years old, proud of it too, my daughters are 25 and 28. I have three grand children, ages 10 and 11 and my youngest grandchild, who was just born August 8, 2006. These children are all, blessings in my eyes, heart and soul. Being able to see them and spend time with them means everything in the world to me. I have a wonderful girlfriend her name is Sharrie, she has been very supportive. She has truly been a blessing to me in so many ways. She has provided me with not only companionship, but also uplifting support with this last breast cancer. She stayed right beside me in the hospital room night and day, and with other surgeries that followed.

There was always so much information to read over. Consent forms, and medications to avoid, which was three pages long. To receive papers on top of papers filled with, all kinds of instructions on the before and after surgery care, describing alternative medication treatments, Risks of skin grafts surgery, Bleeding, and infections, itching and what to do. The inability to heal, Skin scarring, Donor Site Scars, Skin sensations, Skin sensations, Skin contour irregularities, delayed healing, Color changes, Inability to restore function, Surgical anesthesia, this list of information went on and on for pages, and in detail. How can a person not feel intimidated by all of this? I needed someone around all the time. This made the recovery less challenging. To awaken in pain to see one caring person, a loved one, in a cot next to me and to overhear in the dark her silent whispering of prayers for me helped me. Giving me the energy to push harder, to feel that type of stable support when I was ready to give up from the awful stabbing pain, meant everything.

I started feeling worn-out from the continuous tenderness my body needed to recover from through out my torso, tired of the pulling of the six drainage tubes that were surgically attached to my body and slowly growing less interested in fighting. There were those long days and even longer night, of being uncomfortable every moment. Creating an emotion of needing and wanting to have a break from myself, which if you can imagine was very trying to my spirit. Imagine wanting to get away from yourself. Having her right there to distract me made a great difference, taking the focus off of myself. This support was different she made sure I wasn't stressed. I did not have this type of support with the last two battles with breast cancer. This support went both ways, through some intense and persistent communication we worked the difficult times out together. We were committed to hold each other up, when the other person was down, worn out or frustrated. If I said I needed my bedroom painted a soothing color, or to place the furniture in a way to create a positive atmosphere, she made it happen, even if she had to do it all on her own. When I arrived home from the hospital, my bedroom was a beautiful soft color, with new lamps, and brightly colored bedspreads and linen to comfort my spirit. Unfortunately, I could see she was very tired but from all of attempts to contribute to a healthier recovery for me. I was grateful and exceedingly content in my new bedroom. She showed her support in so many different ways. I hope and pray that I live long enough so that I can only return the favor in some great way to show my gratitude.

Three times! I know that there are others, fighting cancer for the third time so how can I sit thinking I should scream out my feelings? There maybe one person out there wondering how they are going to make it through their illness and struggles, needing to hear my story. When I reflect back on the pain and struggles, with the battles of my health issues, and all the different opinions within the family throughout the years, while raising a family and trying to keep my home running was so challenging. I realize and understand that I deserve to express myself. The worries of not having enough funds to replace the washer and dryer or repair the problems in this house such as the large leaky pipes in the basement, a heater that should have been replaced, a broken electric stove, a refrigerator going bad, the sky light in the bathroom that blew away on a snowy day, allowing the rain to coming in on those hard stormy days, although I had the opening covered with Plexiglas, through the crumbling walls and ceiling in the bathroom.

On top of the much needed repairs to the walls in the garage that were falling in with soft dust like substance, with the slightest touch of the hand. The garage door is stuck off of the hinges and completely dry rotted. Like other things that can go wrong in a home that needed immediate attention long ago. Foreclosures and unpaid loans against the house created way before I lived there were strong signs to let go of my grandparent's home. Knowing the house alone was enough to make me want to give up, and at the same time filled with the enough memories to make me feel protected and watched over, giving me strength. The house offered so much and took so much away too. I was killing myself trying to hold on to memories of family members long gone.

I was afraid of a feeling of failing the family, losing something special to all of us. But my hands were tied, being sick, unable to work and disabled.

The doctors instruct me over and over again, not to lift anything over five pounds. With no washer or dryer I needed to go to the laundry mat. So there I was lifting and pulling against doctors orders. Knowing the damages that stress can cause me with my health conditions. The house I am living in was my grandparent's. When they passed away I moved in to help the family but shortly after cancer showed up in me, changing everything.

I was afraid to say I just couldn't manage the house after that, confirming the reality of my situation. I did not want to let everyone down. Not having enough money to pull the load I chose to take on was overwhelming. Fighting for my life has taken all the energy I had left right out of me. Knowing that there are young children fighting cancer, and they have not started living their lives and experience life as I have, almost made me feel, my story was not worth telling. But we are all special and as individuals we should tell our stories and express ourselves because believe it or not the stories are different, as are the experiences.

Well, I don't think I am so special or anything close, but fighting cancer is very special accomplishment. For that reasons alone I continued on with my writing. There is nothing easy about the battle or the recovery. I just took it one step at a time until I was past the treatment and on to the next.

I just want to express my cancer experiences, in hopes that it helps someone who is going through what I have been though, and feeling alone in their struggles.

Each time I finished chemotherapy or radiation treatment and all of the testing required, I would say to myself and anyone listening "I will not do this again." Every time I am faced with this challenge, it takes more away from me and leaves me with less of myself, emotionally and physically. All my life I've had the worse premenstrual cycles. PMS was awful for me . . . But menopause!

The unexpected thing was when Menopause became a major part in my recovery, brought on by the hysterectomy. Menopause alone is a nightmare all on it's on. Bringing on migraine and nausea, keeping me miserably sick from head to stomach, unable to move and enjoy life. Menopause was another side affect acquired during the third breast cancer in 2006, a serious prevention against another cancer. That's another battle in itself, right then when the estrogen was completely out of my body. I didn't know who I had become. It felt like I was in turmoil over night. I know I can be a little dramatic but seriously over night! Now I am left with less of a libido, and more farther from feeling like a complete woman, experiencing a life long numbness throughout my torso. No, I am a complete woman I'm just a different person all together. Starting all over again changing all the time trying hard to figure out who Marnita is, learning what she likes and doesn't like with each passing moment. The normal things change to something new. One negative word or look can make a major difference in my mood that would hurl me into an emotional fit. I end up fighting myself about a world of nothing, with desperation of holing on to my normal way of doing things and suddenly with the aid of medicine from my doctor, like Zanax, Wellbutrin, or Effexor, I was better. Doctors try hard to not wanting to give you Zanax. Every month I fight for it and I am still closely watched with the medication. I do not mind because I have been through so much that, I believe I should have whatever works to keep me balanced. My menopause is pulling on me in so many ways, making it hard to even express the affects I felt inside. Females should not have to go through this, on top of everything else. It's really not fare. I understand it's different from one person to the next, but after the surgeries and all that I am already trying to get used to, menopause is just too much!

I'm not sure what a manic depressant person feel like but I would describe going through full blown menopause as being the same. I was out of control! With the help Zanax I was able to balance out emotionally and began to embrace the changes accruing within my own mind, body and spirit. For years I would fight against taking these medications. Thinking there was nothing wrong with me but, my body was defiantly changing, and I had been naturally fighting the emotional signs for a long time. Listen take the medication, you need it! Your body needs it! Your mind needs it! Even if you don't know you need it! When you feel leveled out, try to eliminate stress from your life because you don't want to stay on the medication forever. You only need it as a crutch then slowly get off of them . . . you can do it! Just don't try to explain menopause to anyone who is nowhere near "The change of life" because they will not understand it nor the noticeable affects it has on you, and that alone will cause you great levels of stress and extreme discomfort. And that will make you feel like you are crazy!

Preserving my life with these preventative treatments against cancer caused me to lose a big portion of my identity. I became fragile, unsure of myself, sensitive, timid, and passive most times. Passive, Oh no, not me passive! Unable to communicate my point of view, that's not me either! I have lost a little more of Marnita than I care to admit. Not ever wanting to get out of bed or to look at myself in the mirror. Try to imagine not wanting to look at yourself in the mirror. Can anyone understand what I am saying? Unable to take medication for Menopause with hormones in them, was a big problem! Estrogen, a female doesn't even know how important estrogen is until it's gone. I needed some hormones real bad! I was screaming for someone to save me, please! I had to change my intake, such as my eating and drinking habits. I had to stay away from the "whites" do less caffeine, chocolates, sugar, soda or liquor, anything that causes change to your system. Stay away from it! My sociable glass of wine here and there became less than sociable. I really needed to keep decaffeinated coffee and herbal tea in the house. This really made the difference in me physically. I was addicted to all of the good stuff. But I needed to keeping my body a little more balanced then off balanced. My Oncologist explained it to me saying that my Menopause was going to be real bad because it was brought on chemically. Meaning if my body was going through "the change of life" naturally, my body would have had a chance to adjust to the lack of hormones it was losing.

With the reconstructive surgery for my new breasts, at the time I didn't care about details, such as the pain levels, or how my nipples were going to be recreated once they were removed, or recovery time. I should have paid closer attention to those details, and asked questions like how long would I need to live with drainage tubes coming out of my body after being released from the hospital and when will I be able to sleep comfortably without using six pillows? As of today I am still healing and I am still uncomfortable. A little bit inpatient trying too hard to get back to the old Marnita. I am grateful for being alive, living and breathing having the gifted to see another day, learning the new Marnita everyday! It just takes a long time to adjust to the newness of things.

There is something you should know about the description of pain levels. It goes like this. The doctors and nurses measure your pain using a scale of 0-10. 0—no pain, 1-3 mild pain-6 moderate and 7-10 sever pain. The surgeon described the pain level as a ten. I understood that, but what I didn't understand is the way 10 feels. I did not know ten-meant unbearable, incomprehensible pain! I would say the pain level was 20 or more, way off the charts for me. I describe the pain as if I was in a terrible car accident unable to remember anything about the incident, being revived soon after the crash. After seven hours of surgery, my family said, when they finally had the chance to see me, I put them out! I thought it was a joke or something because I did have any memory of doing that either. My sister flew all the way here from Georgia and I put them out of my hospital room. I really did not remember at the time. They were trying to see my new body before I had the chance, while I was in so much pain. In my recovering state of mind, I was able to remember them lifting my hospital gown to see my new stomach, excited and happy for me. I guess the pain was so great that I wanted to be alone with it in order to adjust. Looking back at it now, it all appeared to be a dream, coming out of the influence of anesthesia, and some very strong pain medication.

My aunt was 42, with her long secret, losing her battle with breast cancer. She was living in an apartment with (my other aunt) her sister. She wasn't married nor did she have any children. I don't know how or why she was on the floor, but I looked on as the paramedics were trying hard to make her comfortable. I could see her eyes were fixed, locked in a way that I've never seen before. She looked as if she wanted to say something. She couldn't speak and I wondered what she would have said in that moment "I am sorry or I can't do this any more", while looking in my direction. Without blinking, she was letting go, face relaxed and calm. I don't think she wanted to let go, but I believed knowing what I know now it was easier. At some point in all of this, a person has to say stop, question themselves, wondering how much can one person endure, and secretly. I know I've wagered the question of, how bad do I really want to stay to see what life still has to offer me? I understand the feeling but, you must fight and try hard to be strong.

This was going to be my year. My children are grown and really doing well, on their own. I can move on now. I am ready. Having a new grandchild and so many wonderful blessings of support has me, helped me to hold on a little longer, which has been every encouraging. I've taken the genetics test.

The letter

Dear Ms. Kidd-Love

The following letter provides you with a summary of the information we discussed during our appointment when you received the results of your genetic testing. Please feel free to contact me at the following number, with any questions you may have regarding any information contained in this letter or in the information packet you received. Please feel free to have your family members contact me with any questions they may have also.

As we discussed, you were found to have a BRCA1 mutation. This specific mutation that you inherited is called 5502delC. The mutation in your family seems to have come from the maternal side of your family and may be responsible for increased cancer risks in those who inherit the mutation.

The BRCA genes are dominant susceptibility genes. Everyone has two copies of them (BRCA 1 and 2) when they are born. However, some people may be born with a mutation in one of these genes that will make one of the copies not function and therefore they may be more likely to develop a cancer during their lifetime than someone who was born with two normal copies of the genes. Additionally, a parent who is born with a mutation in a BRCA 1 or 2, gene has a 50% chance of passing the gene on to each of their off springs. Men as well as women can pass the gene along to a child and men and women can inherit the mutation in a BRCA gene. The BRCA gene mutations do **NOT** skip generations. This means that if a child does not inherit a BRCA mutation from you, they cannot pass it on to their children.

There are many known increased lifetime risks associated with an inherited BRCA 1 mutation. These are listed in the table and have been compiled from data from the international Breast Cancer Linkage Consortium and The University of Pennsylvania patient population. The table lists the average lifetime for BRCA 1 mutation carriers without any interventions of developing cancer. It is important to note that there are many interventions that have been found to significantly reduce these risks.

As noted there are many options for women today with the BRCA1 mutation. You are a 44-year old woman who was diagnosed with your first breast cancer at 32 and your second breast cancer at 35. Your breast cancers are estrogen and progesterone negative and they are also HER2 negative. You had a recurrence of your breast cancer at the age of 43. You have now had bilateral mastectomies and reconstruction. You will have many options available to you to decrease your risk of developing another cancer. Your doctor and I discussed these options with you, they include: Intensive surveillance and prophylactic surgery. Many people may choose to combine these options of use the along a continuum. Additionally, many may choose to adopt a healthier lifestyle as a means of decreasing their risk of developing cancer.

Increased surveillance is monitoring that detects cancer at the earliest stage possible and when cure is the greatest. Although you have had bilateral mastectomies, there is residual breast tissue and skin that requires an examination. I would recommend that you receive a clinical breast examination every six months if you are not already doing so.

Prophylactic surgeries are to remove organs that have a high risk of developing cancer. Women with BRCA mutations often consider prophylactic bilateral salphingo-oopherectomy, with or without a total hysterectomy. You verbalized that you are very seriously considering this as an option. You stated that you would be discussing this with your gynecologist, and your breast surgeon. It is still possible to develop a breast cancer by as much as 50%, with the removal of your ovaries. This medical team and my self are available to assist in any way possible as well. You have stated that you have completed childbearing and that you were very motivated to pursue this surgical option.

1. Consideration of prophylactic oopherctomy for women beyond child bearing years with a mutation.
2. Consideration of the surveillance clinical trail for family members.

I hope that you will feel free to contact me at any time with questions and that any other family members can call me as well for information and support. Again, my number is attached. I hope that I have been helpful and informative during this process. It has been a pleasure speaking with you. I also ask that you continue to keep in contact with the Cancer Center and inform me if there are any changes in your health status or your family's hearth status. Please notify me if you change your address or phone number also. By doing so, you can be notified if there are any new developments in this area of science.

Please let me know when you would like to participate in research for the University of Pennsylvania. The research would involve contributing three tubes of blood and answering a questionnaire. This research contributes to the ongoing science and may or may not benefit you directly. It will be done at the Rosenfeld Cancer Center. I will forward a copy of this letter with your results to your doctors as you have requested. Please provide me with the names and address of your primary care physician and I will forward a copy there as well.

Thank you for participating in the program. I hope it has been helpful to you. Please let me know if there is anything I can assist you or with.

Sincerely,

Oncology Clinical Nurse Specialist
Breast and Ovarian Cancer Risk Program

Okay long story short. The test came back positive! This was very upsetting to discover. Knowing for sure that I have a mutation gene called BRCA1, and to think that there is a chance that I've passed it on two my daughters.

Taking the genetics test for my children and family was needed, but for me the results made me feel overwhelmed and anxious. I began making copies of my test for everyone in the family. And then to make sure the cancer had not spread, a hysterectomy was the next preventative. Talking about cancer with your family, and taking the genetics are very important ways of prevention. Sit your family down and have them talk about anything and everything concerning your illness. Having cancer was not, just about me, it is about any one carrying our genes. I am sure if my family talked more about cancer in the past, I would have eliminated or monitored my stress by not staying in a mentally and physically abusive marriage. At least I would have created better life habits such as eating healthier, incorporating a healthier lifestyle in every way, from the start.

Knowing you have a gene that causes cancer can offer you a head start on other types of early prevention such as eliminating any use of any and all hormone medication, starting from an early age, especially during my pregnancy. I wouldn't have taken any method of contraceptive using birth control pills, or pre-menopausal medication with a hormone added, even watching stress levels even exercising on a regular.

Learning to eat organic foods may even lessen the chances of reoccurrence. I would have fed my children in a different way using natural ingredients when making their meals. I believe knowing that this means you life, having this knowledge could have helped me. I get to know that I will be fighting, watching and waiting for another battle, until it sneaks up and wins. Thinking I had the gene was one thing but knowing has proved to be totally different.

I know reaching out to strangers, by means of support groups, Internet access, or otherwise, just to have understanding in the fact that the changes, treatments, and anxiety, I am experiencing in my battles are normal is hard to believe, but trust me it helps! You must reach out! It's normal to feel over whelmed, frightened and in shock. If you are in doubt concerning anything, use the internet and Google whatever it is you want to learn on your own.

With the third breast cancer battle, I was in shock to find that technology was further along. The doctors need to find a better way to biopsy a lump in the breast. I cannot understand how the doctors intend on sticking a large long needle into my breast and withdraw fluid. While I am awake! Again! This is 2006. There has to be a better way! I remember standing in the bathroom, looking in the mirror after the chemotherapy treatments started taking my hair out, feeling all alone and exposed, in my darkness with this on going illness.

I wanted to know who this person was staring back at me in the mirror. No way, this can't be me? I was thinking to myself. My hair is long and black and my eyebrows are shaped nice, out lining my eyes, just like my dark lashes. She has a nice face. I don't recognize the girl that mirror, staring back at me, but just in case I better keep an eye on her. She looks like a new canvas waiting, wishing, for something, anything, just to be completed. I have been watching that girl for eight years now.

I've faced this battle a little different this time, having understanding and knowledge. I believe it is not only faith but also the type of support standing beside me. I was able to take photos of my new self, and walk outside without covering my baldness. My baldness is a symbol, a badge of some sort. A life accomplishment badge of honor! You become a soldier in your fight. I really had to face all of my financial issues head on realizing I was not doing a great job holding down the fort. Things just spiraled out of control, not being able to deal with the fact that I had this gene, being sensitive to everything, while knowing that I needed to focus in order to survive. I found myself in a financial rut! Depression started to set in, feeling as if I was constantly losing a battle not with the breast cancer but myself. I was losing because my body was out of control and the bills were behind and pilling up again!

The Linda Creed Breast Cancer Foundation was a rope being thrown into the quicksand of life for me, with my second battle. They helped me financially. I was able to breathe a little better and feel some sense of mental and spiritual peace, when they came to my rescue. I just wanted to thank The Linda Creed Breast Cancer Foundation for being an out reach source for me when I really needed help and had nowhere to turn.

Determined to return to work after completing the second breast cancer, I started feeling tired to the point of not being able to climb the stairs, without breathing hard. I realize I had passed out on my bed, holding a basket of clean laundry. I decided to drive myself to my hospitals emergency room. It was the middle of night a nice, quiet and peaceful trip to the hospital, a little too peaceful when I think about the drive. I found the emergency room empty that evening. I walked right in and received prompt service. That night I learned my heart was slowing down, preparing to stop, not to be resuscitated. My heart became 20% functional. Today I make jokes about me and my 20, saying things like "I was out all day just me and my 20", but it's not funny really, but it keeps my spirit up.

Thanks to the chemotherapy. I will not return to work, which is not good for me, I love working. I could not comprehend this information. A social worker was sent in to my hospital room to explain, and complete forms for my Social Security Disability. Getting over empty nest syndrome was hard enough. Up until this point in my life I was never ever really alone, there were always this kids or someone.

I believe the system should have been set up a little better for any cancer patients, who needs plenty of medication and are not at the age, where they would qualify for most medical coverage. I am not afraid to fight cancer and I am not afraid to die. It seems as if it is going to be a peaceful journey. A journey, I can wait a little longer to take. I hope to encourage other people to hold on and fight a little harder. I want them to know that it is not always going to be easy, and no matter what, we should fight! I will continue to fight! I feel comfortable saying I am a cancer worrier.

I am unable to be a donor, but I can donate my experiences and do my part to help in another way. To share my experiences with those who also feel offended or shocked to see even in this time and age, that these seemingly antiquated treatments are unbelievable normal, and necessary.

Going back, I have tried to think of a time when I felt more like a victim due to my health issues and the things that come to mind at this moment, are the feelings associated with menopause, being financially impotent and the lack of prescription coverage. Menopause really took affect of my entire spirit, even controlling my daily actions amplifying my depression and concerns. People think Menopause is mental and it has challenged me emotionally, causing depression to take on a higher level, which would appear mental to mentally, those who will not or have not experienced it, will think you need a psychologist or something close to that.

Pre-menstrual syndrome for me was bad, but this was extreme. Disabling me physically to the point of not being able to get out of bed nor go out and be around people. I love being around people, helping, comforting and speaking to people came very easy. Suddenly, being sociable became impossible, making me question the thoughtless, normal ways of life as I have been living it, feeling insecure and exposed. Unable to protect myself in simple situations became questionable. Even playful words that I normally would laugh at began to hurt me emotionally.

I could not handle a joke. Not even from my own children. A trip to the supermarket alone was out of the question. I felt overwhelmed and anxious. The Doctor informed me that Menopause is going to be bad, because I was chemically thrown into it, due to Chemotherapy. I am told when you inter Menopause naturally it would not be as bad. Well, that doesn't help me at all. All of this was just words a doctor tells a patient, until I started to really experience changes within myself that I could not explain or describe. I am known as being a beautiful, very sociable, and strong, an aggressive fighter, who finds her own way to get what she needs done. Surviving most difficult situations, not really showing fear only very strong faith. I am older now and being menopausal keeps me waiting on balance, normalcy. The best word that fits me this moment is "fragile".

I had to figure out which medications to take in my little blue bag of medicine. Figuring out which combination of medicine can give me a feeling of balance. Through trial and error this took time. Hormone therapy is totally out of the question, because of my history with breast cancer. Anything with hormones in it is out of the question. I needed control right away!

I have a bag of medicine for the congestive heart failure, such as anxiety, depression, menopause and pain medication from all of my surgeries, dealing with cancer, plastic surgery for the reconstructive breast cancer surgery. Plastic surgery is not the way they show it on television. This is an on going process, of corrections that take place until you are happy with the finished product. I was unaware of the lengthy time it takes to complete breast with nipples and tattoos. Taking time to figuring out what medication worked well with the other medicine for pain control and constipation that started with the pain medicine, while desperately searching for a happy medium in order to feel as if I weren't on any medication all became very important.

Repeating plastic surgery in order to make my breast appear normal in my clothes was all I really wanted and needed. Having stability and control once again in my life became a prioritized goal achievement plan. Working hard with my team of physicians, and exercise instructors in order to feel healthy again was what I needed to feel in control of my life first.

Not forgetting that I had a home, car and bills that I needed to stay on top of. Making decisions to buy food for the house or medicine that my heart needs everyday is a difficult choice. Especially when you have the so called understanding bill collectors ringing your phone and standing at your door demanding small payments such as three and four hundred dollar checks that you really don't have threatening to turn off your energy supply. Chemotherapy for me was given intravenously by way of a port in my chest, above the breast. The treatment took between three to four hours to administer.

Once, I was given Benadryl, which caused me to experience crazy feet, or restless leg syndrome. I couldn't keep my legs from moving. Getting out of my chair with my intravenous pole was the only way to get past the feeling of (R.L.S) restless leg syndrome. I needed to move around, and walk about the unit. I grew hatred for the red fluid being pumped into my veins. The taste left in my mouth was metallic. It took days to flush the taste out of my mouth. I couldn't help thinking I was able to smell the red poison, made to kill off the active cells, infected or not with cancer in my body, whenever I took a breath I felt the sent of chemotherapy was in the air. If I make that first phone call to get things started, this is all going to go so fast and I will not know what happened to the time.

I know that Doctors have their reasons for telling you just enough information and not all, unless you know to ask, but this discovery was pertinent information that should have been brought to my attention from my Oncologist before the treatments began, knowing there is a chance of Congestive Heart Failure as a recurring side affect that occurs in a moderate percentage of people with chemotherapy treatment. Not knowing anything about the HPV virus. My Gynecologic Oncologist explained to me that a normal healthy female can fight off this virus, but my body can not because my immune system has been weakened with all of the cancer treatments, therefore a Hysterectomy was needed, right away. It's now 2006 and I am 44, soon to be 45years old on March 22, 2007. My daughters are 25 and 28 years old. I have three grand children ages 10 and11 and my youngest grandchild, just born August 8, 2006. I have a wonderful partner who is very supportive.

She has provided me with not only companionship, but also uplifting support with this last breast cancer. She stayed right beside me in the hospital room night and day. This made the battle less challenging. To awaken in pain and see a caring person in a cot next to me, and to overhear in the dark her silent whisper of prayers for me, helped me to feel that sound stable support when I was ready to give up from the stabbing pain, tired of hurting and fighting. It made a difference for me, because I did not have that type of support with the last two battles of breast cancer.

With my second battle with cancer I was dating a girl who wasn't able to see me go through the effects of breast cancer and she was a nurse. So we agreed to separate as friends. There were other female friends but you need unconditional love that goes both ways in order to deal with something so great, and this is the type of support I have now. This is support that goes both ways, we worked together, holding each other up when the other person is down. No threats of being left alone any more. Three times! I know that there are others, fighting cancer for the third time so how can I sit thinking I should scream out my feelings. When I sit and reflect back on the pain and struggles of this battle, and trying to keep my home running. I realize and understand that I deserve to express myself.

The worries of not having enough funds to take replace or repair the problems like a broken electric stove, refrigerator, the sky light in the bathroom blew away allowing the rain to coming in on those hard stormy days, on top of the basement walls falling in like dust with the softest touch of the hand and the garage door is stuck off of the hinges and completely dry rotted. Like other things that can go wrong in a home that need immediate attention long ago. Seeing people on talk shows, talking about their experiences with cancer and knowing that there are young children fighting cancer, and they have not started living their lives and experience life like I have, almost made me feel, my story is not worth writing. But we are all special and as individuals we should tell our stories and express ourselves because, believe it or not the stories are different as well as the experiences.

Well, I did not think that I was special enough to tell my story, but fighting cancer is very special giving me the experience to teach and inform other who are waking up to the same nightmare needing the comfort of knowing that there is someone who understands the pain and suffering they may experience in their treatment. I want to say to that person that there is nothing easy about this, but being a fighter means everything! I just want to express my cancer experiences, in hopes that it helps someone who is going through what I have been though, and feels alone in their struggles.

At the time of reconstruction surgery I did not care about details, such as the pain level, how my nipples were going to be recreated once they were removed, or how long it would take for my body to completely heal. The only thing I cared about at the time was having perky breasts and a flat stomach, so I can get into that two piece bathing suit. I should have asked questions like how long would I need to live with the drainage tubes coming out of my body after being released from the hospital and when will I be able to sleep comfortably without using six pillows? As of today I am still healing and I am still in some pain. Of course, I am grateful for being here, living and breathing another day, learning the new me. People tell me all the time, that I look so healthy. They find it hard to believe that I was ever sick.

My Oncologist said that he wished half of his patients looked as good as I looked. I was always headstrong and full of energy.

Having an "I can do it" attitude all of my life. Being independent, and being in control was always very important to me. It was nothing for me to be the head of my little family. Always, ready to listen, help, and try to resolve problems of my friends or family. But I started to feel run down. I started experiencing less and less energy as the days passed. One evening I was bringing up a load of laundry from the basement, I began to realize that my shortness of breath was getting worse, when climbing the stairs, a simple task, which became physically impossible to do. I was told I had Bronchitis and was taking medicine for that for weeks, which was not helping at all. I was still finding it difficult to breath. My chest continued to feel tight. I remember making it to the top of the stairs, after washing clothes. I felt tired and short of breath walking down the hallway towards my bedroom, placing the basket down and sitting on the edge of my bed. What I could not remember was lying back. I had passed out in the sitting position, with my legs touching the floor. I realized then that I needed to go to the emergency room and right away! But, I did not want to go to any hospital. I wanted to go to my own hospital, where everyone knew me. So, I drove myself to the hospital emergency room, still that thinking I had Bronchitis. Arriving to the emergency room alone, I began to explain to the nursing staff at the sign in window, that I was having trouble catching my breath. They quickly placed me into a wheelchair and hooked me up to monitors that checked my pulse and heart rate, while they took my history and inter my information into the computer as quickly as they could.

That was the fastest service I had ever encountered from an emergency room visit. I found it funny because I did not think I was that sick for all that much attention. They took blood several times and found out that my heart was slowing down. It was explained to me, that my heart was slowing down to stop and not to be resuscitated. I was admitted into the hospital not even aware that I was on the Intensive Care Unit, of Abington Memorial Hospital until I was being wheeled out of my room for extended testing. I could see in the hallway some serious medical equipment and my Pastor running down the unit asking for me. No body from St. Peters church knew anything about me being in the hospital. How did she know because I didn't even know how serious my health was, but that's when everything slowed down and stopped! It was as if I had all of a sudden awakened from what already felt like a dream. I was later diagnosed with another deficiency called Congestive Heart Failure, not only did my heart expand with clots, but I also had fluid in my lungs due to the chemotherapy treatments. The hospital had to send a social worker into my room to explain that I would not be going back to work and that she was filling out forms for my Social Security Disability. I was in the hospital for twelve days wondering how I was going to make it, not being able to return to work. Talking about feeling overwhelmed. My mind just could not grasp on to this new information.

I know that Doctors have their reasons for telling you just enough information and not all, unless you know to ask, but this discovery was pertinent information that should have been brought to my attention from my Oncologist before the treatments began, knowing there is a chance of Congestive Heart Failure as a recurring side affect that occurs in a moderate percentage of people with chemotherapy treatment.

Doctors should inform their patients that the likelihood of these cancer treatments may show side affects such as congestive heart failure. Breast cancer is no stranger to my family. My family members that experienced it have passed on. They did not believe in talking about "cancer", they tried hard to keep it quiet. It was kept a secret, until they could not hide it anymore. The cancer was taking them away from the family, removing them out of our lives. I believe we should talk about cancer. Leave notes, journals and photos expressing the harsh reality of cancer. Now, I need all of my energy to focus on myself. Learning to stay positive and taking note to what is important and what is not. Restricting myself to resolving my own problems became a challenge. Being unaware, and not having any guidance from my mother, who won her battle twice with her breast cancer, ending up with Congestive Heart Failure herself, unable to stop working she passed away with an aneurisms, while attending a church meeting.

My father tells me that my mother and I shared the same afflictions, which makes me wonder, what is next. My youngest aunt (my mothers sister) lost her battle with breast cancer at an early age, and then my grandmother who suffered with pancreas cancer, are all gone now leaving me alone and in the dark about the changes and reactions my body was going to experience from the much needed treatments. These treatments as harsh as it may seem, were by the book procedures that caused me to mentally feel secluded from the world?

When my life took a turn for the worse, I was not mentally prepared for it, but when you think of life and its experiences, are any of us ready for it? I believe things happen for a reason. Having my children when I did as a teenager was meant to be, I wasn't ready but I made the best of it. I realized now having my children when I did was the right choice. If I had waited I don't think I would have had the energy to get through the three breast cancers, related congestive heart failure, hysterectomy, and Menopause, while raising my two children as a single parent. Being single at the time and getting over empty nest syndrome was hard enough. I wanted to return to work, and get on with my life. It's been a long struggle raising two daughters and trying to keep up as if I had help from my ex-husbands, their father. Doctors visits, dental visits, hair dressers appointments, school clothes and supplies, parent teachers meetings, entertainment and food shopping, school trips, making sure they were safe ever second of the day, all of their needs fell on me, alone.

Being a single parent is heavy stress all in it's self. Living with cancer I am able to say, I am not afraid to fight cancer and I am not afraid to die. I'm blessed and I know I'll be okay no matter what happens having faith and believing in Gods will, also thinking back to the time when my heart was slowing down to stop. It seems as if it is going to be a peaceful journey. At the same time a journey, I can wait a little longer to take never the less. I hope to encourage other people to hold on and fight a little harder.

I want them to know that it is not always going to be easy, and no matter what, even if it takes prevention, we should fight back! I will continue to fight! Going back, I have tried to think of a time when I felt like a victim due to my health issues and the only thing that comes to mind at this moment, are the feelings associated with menopause, battling to have prescription coverage, the lack of understanding from close love ones, resulting to standing in rain, snow and heat while weak long lines waiting on free food. Menopause really took affect of my entire spirit, even controlling my daily actions. People think Menopause is mental, but it challenged me emotionally, causing depression to take on a higher level, which would appear mental to those who will not or have not experienced it. Pre-menstrual syndrome for me was bad, but this was worse. Disabling me physically to the point of not being able to get out of bed nor go out and be around people. I love being around people, helping, comforting and speaking to people I did not know came very easy. Suddenly, being sociable became impossible, making me question the thoughtless, normal ways of life as I have been living it, feeling insecure and exposed. Unable to protect myself in simple situations became questionable. Even playful words that I normally would laugh at began to hurt me emotionally. I could not handle a joke. A trip to the supermarket alone was out of the question. I felt overwhelmed and anxious. I walked into the market one day, picking up everything I needed. When it was time to pay for my groceries I started to feel an anxiety attack.

Needless to say I walked right out of the market leaving the entire cart of food standing in the isle. I just didn't know how to ask for help, because I didn't know I needed help, so when it wasn't offered I would force myself to move past all of these negative emotions that stripped me of my independence. The Doctor informed me that Menopause is going to be worse because I was chemically thrown into it, due to Chemotherapy. I am told when you inter Menopause naturally it would not be as bad. Well, that doesn't help me at all. All of this was just words a doctor tells a patient, until I started to really experience changes within myself that I could not explain or describe.

Repeating plastic surgery to make my breast appear normal in my clothes is one of the things I needed to work on in order to take control of my life first. Looking as normal as I could for myself was important. Not forgetting that I had a home, car and other bills that I needed to stay on top of, making decisions to buy food for the house or medicine that my heart needs everyday is a difficult choice. I found myself constantly wishing I had somebody close to me to explain what was ahead of me.

Carrying this illness made me feel alone just having the skin on my breast completely burn off from the radiation treatments which was painful in itself. I mean how in the world do you put a bra or shirt over raw skin? Not to mention the loss of hair and that includes eyebrows and other unmentionable places. Getting back to work was always on my mind. I had family responsibilities, long over due debts to deal with, and a house to run. Ready to return to work with only a few more radiation treatments to go, everything looks good, so I thought it was anyway. Who in the world wants to get back to work?

That should tell you something about the job I had. I enjoyed going to work. I was a Bursar for Temple University, collecting money owed from patients, Insurance companies on unpaid accounts. Getting dressed for work, feeling like an independent, modern day working female, was good for me, this is what I was comfortable doing everyday. I was proud, having my own office and great responsibilities handling large amounts of money everyday. I had respect and trust. Of course I was bonded, and took my job seriously. This time I had a Trams Flap surgery. The procedure is a double mastectomy and reconstructive surgery, where they used muscles from my stomach and created new breast with those muscles. From what I understand they replace the stomach muscles with a band from a cadaver.

Well, I have nice size "c" cups and a beautiful flat stomach, which I have always dreamed, of having after having two babies. The plastic surgeon (which I am truly grateful for) assured me that I would be able to have a flat stomach, as an incentive of losing my breasts. I was so happy, thinking that there was a brighter side to this pain, I was about to encounter. At the time did not care about details, such as the pain level, how my nipples were going to be recreated once they were removed, or how long it would take for my body to completely heal. I should have asked questions like how long would I need to live with these drainage tubes coming out of my body after being released from the hospital and when will I be able to sleep comfortably without using six pillows?

As of today I am still healing and I am still in pain, feeling much discomfort. Don't get me wrong, of course, I am grateful for being here, living and breathing another day, learning the new me. There is something you should know about describing pain levels. It goes like this. The doctors and nurses measure your pain using a scale of 0-10. 0—no pain, 1-3 mild pain, 4-6 moderate and 7-10 sever pain. The surgeon described the pain level as a ten. I did not know ten-meant unbearable pain. I would say the pain level was 20. I describe the pain as if I was in a terrible car accident unable to remember anything about the incident.

After seven hours of surgery, my family said I put them out of my hospital room. I did not remember at the time. They were trying to see my new body before I had the chance. In my recovering state of mind, I could remember them lifting my hospital gown to see my new stomach, excited and happy for me. Looking back at it now, at the time it all seems like a dream, coming out of the influence of anesthesia.

This was going to be my year. My children are grown and really doing well, on their own. I can move on now. I am ready. Having a new grandchild and a youthful partner standing with me, helped me to hold on a little longer, which has been every encouraging. I've taken the genetics test. The results turned out "positive" Which is not to be great for me. I know for sure that I have a mutation gene called BRCA1. Taking the genetics test for my children and family was needed, but for me the results made me feel overwhelmed, anxious, to make sure the cancer had not spread. A hysterectomy is the next preventative procedure. On top of feeling like a lab rat of some kind, I also get to know that I will be fighting, watching and waiting for another battle, until it sneaks up and wins. Thinking I had the gene was one thing but knowing has proven to be totally different. What a year I am having. I know reaching out to strangers, by means of support groups, Internet access, or otherwise, just to have understanding in the fact that the changes, treatments, and anxiety I am experiencing in my battles are normal is hard to believe, but trust me it helps. You must reach out! The doctors need to find a better way to biopsy a lump in the breast. I cannot understand how the doctors intend on sticking a large long needle into my breast and withdraw fluid. While I am awake! Again! This is 2006. There has to be a better way. I remember standing in the bathroom, looking in the mirror after the chemotherapy treatments started taking my hair out, feeling all alone and exposed, in my darkness with this illness.

I wanted to know, who this person was staring back at me in the mirror. No way, this can't be me? I was thinking to myself. My hair is long and black and my eyebrows are shaped nice, out lining my eyes, just like my dark lashes. She has a nice face. I don't recognize that girl in the mirror, staring back at me, but just in case I better keep an eye on her.

She looks like a new canvas waiting, wishing, for something, anything, just to be completed. I have been watching that girl for eight years now. I've faced this battle a little different this time. I believe it is not only faith but also the type of support standing beside me.

Eight years later and I am still adjusting. I believe the "system" for people who are in need, should be set up a little better for people who are in need for continued care. Cancer patients, who need plenty of medication and are not at the age where they would qualify for most medical coverage, need additional help with medical coverage. In my case I was either too old to enter a program like the "Chip program for children" and too young for Medicare. I was told I received too much money to qualify for welfare, and really I don't get enough money to stay on top of everything. I was rejected all the way around. I am not afraid to fight cancer and I am not afraid to die. It seems as if it is going to be a peaceful journey. All the same a journey I can wait on taking all the same. Even with the increased depression I can still say that's a journey I can wait a little longer to take. With this book, I hope to encourage other people to hold on and fight a little harder. I want them to know that, it isn't always going to be easy, things can get pretty ruff but no matter what, we should fight the cancer that threatens our lives. There has been times when I've said I'm not going to fight another battle, but that wasn't right, to say. I owe it to my children and grandchildren to continue the fight. Catching cancer early is the first thing, also being aware of your body is most important. Identifying any new and sudden changes can save your life!

Going back, I have tried to think of a time when I felt like a victim due to my health issue and the only thing that comes to mind at this moment, are the feelings associated with menopause, being financially impotent and when that was a lack prescription coverage. Menopause really took affect of my entire spirit, even controlling my daily actions. People think Menopause is mental, but it challenged me emotionally, causing depression to take on a higher level, which would appear mental to those who will not or have not experienced it.

Pre-menstrual syndrome was always hard with me, but this was worse. Disabling me physically to the point of not being able to get out of bed nor go out and be around people. I love being around people, helping, comforting and speaking to people I did not know came very easy. Suddenly, being sociable became impossible, making me question the thoughtless, normal ways of life as I have been living it, feeling insecure and exposed. Unable to protect myself in simple situations became questionable. Even playful words that I normally would laugh at began to hurt me emotionally. I could not handle a joke. A trip to the supermarket alone was out of the question. I felt overwhelmed and anxious. The Doctor informed me that Menopause is going to be worse because I was chemically thrown into it, due to Chemotherapy. I am told when you inter Menopause naturally it would not be as bad. Well, that doesn't help me at all. All of this was just words a doctor tells a patient, until I started to really experience changes within myself that I could not explain or describe. I am sometimes known to be beautiful in spirit, very sociable, strong, and an aggressive fighter, who finds her own way to get what she needs done.

Surviving most difficult situations, not really putting much energy in showing my own fears and staying close to my very strong faith, has permitted me to stand strong. I am older now and being menopausal keeps me waiting on balance, normalcy. The best word that fits me this moment is "fragile". I had to figure out which medications to take in my little blue bag of medicine. Figuring out which combination of medicine can give me a feeling of balance. Through trial and error this took time. Hormone therapy is totally out of the question, because of my history with breast cancer. Anything with hormones in it is out of the question. I needed control right away! A doctor once advised me to stay away from any medicine starting with "E" for Estrogen. Although she laughed, I took that advice to heart. I have a bag of medicine for the congestive heart failure, also for anxiety, depression, menopause and pain medication from all of my surgeries, dealing with cancer, plastic surgery for the reconstructive breast cancer surgery. This has become an going process, which I was unaware of, taking time to figuring out what medication worked well with the medicine I was already taking in order to feel as though I weren't on any medication at all became very important to me.

Repeating plastic surgery to make my breast appear normal in my clothes is what I needed to work on first. This would allow me to start taking control of my life again. I felt there was a chance if I didn't like myself on the outside, when I looked in the mirror I wouldn't have been happy and it may have an negative effect on my self esteem. I really couldn't have that. I already had a lot of other stuff pulling me down like my home that needed a lot of work, an old broken down used car and tons of back bills that I needed to get back on top of from the onset of my health issues. On top of trying to decide which was the most important, the bills or my medical needs, I didn't know which end was up. I truly felt helpless. I often wondered if I should buy food for the house or medicine for my heart. All of it became a very difficult choice, depressing me even further, because I needed both. The up coming visit to the Gynecologist was enlightening. Now, the new thing was the HPV virus. Everywhere you turn you hear the concerns of the HPV virus. This is one more thing for females to worry about on top of everything else. My Gynecologic Oncologist explained to me that a healthy female can fight off this virus, but my body couldn't because my immune system had been weakened with all of the cancer treatments. Therefore as a preventative measure a Hysterectomy was needed and right now, to prevent the likely hood of ovarian cancer. It's 2006 and I am now 44 years old, my daughters are 25 and 28. I have three grand children ages 10 and 11 and my youngest grandchild, just born August 8, 2006. I have a wonderful friend, who was the only neighbor to step out of her world and into mine.

Helping me whenever she could, being very supportive. There were only a few people on my block knew of my battles with cancer. Her family didn't know what I was dealing with inside my house all alone. They only knew that my hair was very short all of a sudden, making them wonder. Her family members knew nothing about me or my health issues. I guess they thought that I was crazy cutting off all of my hair. We laugh about it now but I know people really don't care enough to ask if you are okay, and really mean it. If one person can step out of their world with good intent and walk into yours this world would be a much better place. This Neighbor once finding out about my medical history, has provided me with not only companionship, but also uplifting support with this last breast cancer. She offered me much more than a helping hand.

She took time off from work time and time again to sit with me before, during and after surgery. She was and still is a strong light at the end of the tunnel, staying right by my side. In the evenings she slept in my hospital room on a little cot, next to my bed throughout the night. She took on the job of running back and fourth to care for my home, my pets, plants and anything else that needed attention. I really thank God for her. She went beyond being a neighbor and friend. She extended herself as a humanitarian. Handing me hope on a platter, not just with words but in her actions. She put herself out there protecting me, when she could in order to keep negativity, and unnecessary stress away from me. I believe I would have given up this time, if she weren't right there with me this time around.

Having her and a few others from my church made the battle less challenging. Not having someone next to you while you are experiencing great pain, vomiting and discomfort during your recovery, makes it easier to give in to that never ending pain. This way I was able to focus on myself, distracted in such a positive way with a concerned hands holding on to mine. An empathetic heart praying you through it all, you're encouraged to get past it. It's just like having labor pains while in child birth. You need and want someone close to you to help you deliver your baby. There's no difference.

To awaken in pain and see a caring person in a cot in arms reach next to my hospital bed, and to overhear in the dark a whispering prayer, for me was so inspirational. That incredible stable support was exactly what I needed this time, when I was ready to give in to the stabbing pain, and nausea tired of hurting, tired of feeling sick, and tired of fighting. Fighting for comfort, fighting for mental peace, fighting neighbors who are jealous because they don't know why I'm not wasn't running to work like them everyday. They were unable to understand why my yard was a mess or why they see different people stopping over to take my trash out or to trim the trees in the yard for me. Really they didn't care, it's easier to just judge and say hurtful things, instead of showing any real concern for a neighbor.

One little person made a huge difference for me when I was just beginning to wonder what the point was in fighting? I had support with the other battles which was great, but this support was extremely different offering me a greater sense of mental peace unlike the last two battles with breast cancer. I felt as though I was being completely heard. To know someone hears me for once was crucial at that point in my life. Feeling secluded and defeated, I really needed to be heard and I was. It saved my life . . . .

I live with many scars, one's that you can't see from being in a physical and mentally abusive marriage with my ex-husband, the father of my daughters and the scars that are visible, on my body telling the story of how cancer tried it's best to take me away from here. The scars ache and at times itch on rainy days. These scars on my chest where the port use to be and the scar where my new breast were recreated from the lower part of my stomach, all still bother me constantly reminding me of my illness.

Although the areola and nipples look great there are scars around and just below the areola of both breasts. The skin was taken from the lower area of my stomach, little sprouts of hair appear here and there making me feel, less likely to expose my breast, comfortably. My plastic surgeon advised me that he could fix this problem but wasn't able to keep up on my bills from the office visits, which caused me to not go as often as required, for completion of the reconstructive surgery. My breasts still feel as if they don't belong on my body. Keeping me a lot warmer than normal and there is numbness, from my chest to the bottom of my stomach, as if I had on some type of chest armor or a bullet proof vest. The other scar is a large abdominal scar that stretches from one side of my hip to the other. It's in the shape of a smile. I'm getting use to seeing myself but, let me tell you something. I would love to find out where those movie stars go to have their plastic surgery. My surgery, as blessed as I may be looks nothing like theirs.

Well, after a few battles with my recurring illnesses, I had to make some other difficult but necessary decisions realizing that it was time to look after my self. The fact that I have tested positive for the cancer gene and knowing that the last few battles, really took a lot of my energy away, preparing for the next battle come with some serious changes. I've had my hands full with my own life raising two daughters as a single parent from a young age and I need to make some healthy choices concerning the way I would like to live out the rest of my life. For one, that meant cutting the umbilical cord that held me tightly to my grown daughters. This is one huge hurtle for me to achieve, successfully.

Especially, when I feet I was the one holding on to them. They were showing me time and time again that they didn't really need me any more. They had their own lives to live and that was painfully clear to see. When they stopped calling to see if I was okay or in need of something or another, confirmed everything.

They really didn't have the time, not the type of time I felt their disabled mother or any mom should received from her two daughters she raised as a singly. I had to learn the hard way that in some cases this is the way it is . . . . Our children owe us nothing!

With my last surgery, a total hysterectomy a prevention for pancreas cancer, which was a few months after my bi-lateral mastectomy and reconstructive surgery, was more than frightening for me. This time, my daughters, sisters, brother, aunt or uncles showed up to the hospital, until the next day, and later in the afternoon. Even then I had to call them over and over again to see where everyone was, only to see my two daughter's, my three grandchildren and a friend of theirs walked in to my hospital room, giving me the impression of being less concerned and tired of the visiting me after another surgery. As if there was nothing to worry about, because mom was always great, fine or doing well. The sting of their lack of concern hurt leaving me to wonder if anyone actually cared if I lived or died. I know our family members mean well. Sometimes we (as people) just don't think things all the way through. This including myself, I am just as guilty of this as the next person. I was left to feel that feeling of "you've worn out your welcome" you know when you've stayed longer than expected?

I was defiantly worried because after this surgery I suffered with great nausea and vomiting. The doctors explained that this was a reaction to the anesthesia. I had never before, experienced a reaction from the anesthesia. The pain stayed with me all through the night and with no immediate family being there was a little frightening to me. I began to question my existence. I felt the family was taking my illness for granted, thinking as usual that I was all right. This added to my anxiety and depression. I woke up to the reality that they weren't taking my health issues serious as they should. I know I am a survivor but come one . . . I had to call to see where they all were, before I received a visit. What is that all about? When I came home they still didn't have much time for me, calling every once in a while but not coming to give me any real assistance, leaving the care giving to others.

This is my fault I know, because I have always shown to be stronger than the average person. At my age and experiencing the things I had to endure. Always hiding my pain and discomfort away from them, I did not want to scare them into thinking that there mother; sister, aunt or niece was dyeing. That fear kept me wanting to appear stronger than I really was. Making them build up this attitude that I was always okay, even when I really wasn't.

This is a funny story, right after my hysterectomy my daughters stopped over to visit me. This was after they did whatever they had to do earlier that morning. I was informed that they had stuff to do after their visit with me also. This was very frustrating to me because I wanted more than a "visit" from my daughters this time. They came into the house joyfully, being as playful as they are normally with one another. I can hear them coming into the house, below my bedroom, making their way up the stairs, they were all dressed up holding their, fresh cups of coffee in hand. I was upstairs sitting straight up, in my rocking chair, after making my way out of bed. My drainage tubes were pinned to my gown. I prepared for them to, try to make their getaway. I was very determined to get their attention, my hair undone looking a mess, and needing a bath and some other help.

Feeling a little spiteful that morning, when I realized they weren't taking their mothers health serious. I found myself so upset, so I got a little even, deciding to let my good friend and care giver take a break from helping me. Telling her to please go out for the day, because I could see she was not going to make it to the next day. Her energy was beginning to run low. And she still needed to return to work. So, she left the house as I asked. Only to go shopping for, some more house hold goods, so that I could care for myself, when I was alone. We set up my bedroom with a microwave, toaster oven, and a small fridge for convince. That way I wouldn't take on the stairs, trying to get something to eat.

Anyway, back to my story. My daughters could take a chance at doing what she has to do for one day, and see what we had to do just to get my day started. When they approached my bedroom all dressed up looking nice, cheerful as usual. I waited for the question, and then they asked it. They asked me if I needed anything . . . and usually I would say" and let me admit this, I would always say 'as a way of not being a bother or worrying anyone" . . . , "I'm okay" but this time I thought best to answered "yes, I do need help," which surprised me hearing it come from my own mouth. I expressed to them that I needed my hair shampooed and braided and a shower. Well, a shower and shampoo sounds easy right? Not when you have tape and drainage tubes hanging off of your body. There was a lot to it because I was, tremendously sore and bound with after surgery tape and other stuff.

My youngest daughter, at the time pregnant but healthy enough to shampoo her mother's hair, was ready to take on the challenge. After looking at each other for seconds, as you would imagine twin sisters would do, they got to work . . . Pinning up my after surgery drainage tubes and bulbs to the shower curtain, one shampooed while the other bathed me. My bathroom was not big enough for three people, but we worked it out. Now, standing in my tub, they were scrubbing away. My daughters are comfortable seeing me without clothes. For a long time it was just the three of us, or mostly females in the house anyway. But to have to physically wash my person was another thing all together. They washed, scrubbed, and rinsed, until they were out of their nice shirts, hair no longer down and flowing, pulled up into hair ties to protect it from the sweat building up on their body's, now standing there in their bras and bare feet working hard.

My youngest daughter mentioned that she was very tired and she hadn't eaten. You know the feeling you get when coffee hits your stomach and there is no food there to catch it, and she was pregnant at the time? Well, my oldest daughter went rushing off to the kitchen downstairs to make her sister something to eat, while she continued braiding my hair. The truth is I could have shampooed my own hair and taken the time to get a shower but I needed them to see how difficult and time consuming it was to complete the job. My girlfriend "Sharrie" was not only taking care of me by doing that but also answering my door to concerned visitors while showing them up to my room, extending herself bringing all of us something to eat and drink. On top of running my house for me and that included constant care of my pets, a cat, a dog, and all of my plants twenty four hours a day, while she continued to check up on her mother, her own cat and their home.

The damage was already done. My daughters didn't seem to get the message, I wanted them to get. They didn't change their ways by going out of their way to offer any on going care with extra assistance on their own, without me having to ask for the help and I didn't think I had to ask for on going help. I just wanted to be taken care of by them while I had them. So, at least I got a little laugh out of that day, because seeing them work so hard for me was extremely amusing. Especially, seeing the look on my oldest daughters face while she washed those unmentionable places on my body, with her eyes close tight, saying over and over again "it's nothing, this is no different than washing Taylor" her own little daughter. We all broke out laughing, knowing it all looked and felt very funny, because she continued to say "It's nothing different, I'm washing my car" over and over again . . . We laughed so hard. All the while, my youngest daughter is reaching over her in order to shampoo my hair.

I would do it for them and I have, and as a mother you know I have. They're my babies, the only ones I have. I didn't see why they couldn't stop to take care of their mother for a few hours, right? But to see the look on their faces, knowing I could have taken the delicate time to pin my own drainage tubes to the shower curtain and slowly make my way through the morning process of getting up and dressed, wasn't as serious as I had made it out to be was as the commercials say "priceless"! The adventure was very comforting and amusing to see them in action.

Let me explain why I went through all of this with them. I have my reasons, for doing the things I do. I want to tell you why, tricking my daughters into spending that type of quality time, with their mother, was very important to me. Yes, I didn't think they were taking my illness serious enough, we know that but there is another reason.

See my own mother, left out to go to our church one evening for a church meeting and while she was there she had, an aneurism or something like it, the bottom line is she was gone without warning! The point is we really don't know what is going to happen to us, from one day to the next. All I knew was my mother, who I never had the chance to say good bye too or "I love you" and "what do you need me to do for you today" was gone . . .

Just stop and think of all the things you would say to your mother. My mother went to our church home, St. Peters Lutheran Church, like normal and never come home. The last time I saw her she was being placed into an ambulance, not moving at all, on her way to the hospital, where she would never speak another word again. She was not walking out of the church this time she was being carried out on a stretcher! I will never get over that day. And I still attend this church feeling her presence everywhere I sit. Always, dreading days like Mother's Day, or Grandparents Day, knowing that I am both, it's very painful to sit through a sermon. But there is no other place I'd rather be on a Sunday morning. I wish I can touch her, talk to her, hear her voice, enjoy one more flea market, and fight over who saw what first. You know help her in any way possible? If I had that chance, but I can't and it hurts to know this. That is why I had my two daughters stop their busy world to take some time out for, even if they don't understand now, they'll always have the memory of that day with the three of us in that little bathroom together.

My mother kept her battles a complete secret but if I knew my mother was fighting breast cancer I would have been there worried to death about her every need and want, touching her, kissing her, hearing her voice or any thing else out of fear of her possible death. But that's me . . . .

Whenever my daughters need me, and I mean from their birth, as a mother I've always tried to take any and every opportunity to do whatever I could, even now because old habits are hard to break and I love them with all my heart and soul. I am guilty of simply wanting to make things right for them, to the best of my ability, especially while I was able. It is what I was accustomed to doing for my girls. My philosophy at the time was, if I could accomplish little I would try hard to do more for my daughters. You want your children to grow up and move on, but nothing prepares you for the emotions behind the separation. I was happy and extremely sad at the same time. I was happy that they were doing well and sad that they didn't include my wellbeing in their accomplishment. That's life!

We all have our lessons to learn including myself and believe it or not that was a hard lesson for me to accept. Having to fight cancer several times has been the most humbling experienced for me. I have for many years had the appearance of being half of my true age, looking more like my daughters sister than, their mother. I was short, strong but sturdy. My oldest calls me "stumpy" it's a running joke of hers. I've quickly gone from being a strong independent, single super mom with a family, who worked full time at one hospital or another, having a love for strength, exercise and healthiness. I worked part time as a weight lifting instructor at the YMCA in my twenties, or where ever I could to earn extra money to take care of my family. Only to become a dependent person at the age of thirty-five, blessed, but stuck in this body, which looks okay but is very limited physically. Always, feeling and needing some type of "assistance", of the typical eighty year old. Everyday is different for me, and I have my good days which are great! Then there are those bad days. The bad days seem to take a toll on me, pulling me down physically and most importantly emotionally.

There are children who feel they owe the world to their parents. Others leave the nest, never thinking to look back. Most parents dream of that day, waiting for their children to go off to college. I know . . . but I am an empty nest mom. I never imagined my life without my children. Never considered it until I returned from dropping off my youngest daughter off leaving her in her college dorm and realizing there was nobody else to take care of, but myself. Heart breaking! Yes! Fly away from the nest because that is what they are supposed to do. Okay, but don't go too far away. It was always just the three of us.

They flew away and didn't look back. They don't put the effort at least not the same energy I've put into them, when they were growing up and needed me. My children are in the middle of that, looking back but not enough, with the idea of "Oh! Mom's okay". That realization was very heart braking for me to accept. At first then I realized the way I was with my own mother. In my mind she was okay too. I didn't know any better either. After you've struggled to raise your children, you wish for the day they leave home, and then there are other times when you raise them and never want them to leave because they are all you have. I always say "some bad things happen for good". So, maybe it is best, my children are flying on their own making their way through life and aren't attached by their umbilical cords. I would rather them to be strong and able to survive without me, than weak and dependent with their worlds falling apart without me. You just never know what's going to happen . . . .

Just because you don't have what you need, like medicine, or food, don't "expect", your grown children to rush to your side, reaching into their filled cabinets or pockets to send you a safety rope, with thoughts of helping you out. Some children's minds were not thinking that way. Listen, if your children have a family of their own, demanding jobs and are working hard to get through college to earn their degrees. See this is what my daughters were trying to manage and balance in their own lives as single parents. I believe my daughters meant well. We as parents just can't expect our children to automatically know, to do for us. Just don't **expect** anything! **If you do not expect anything you'll be better off.** Your children might surprise you. I believe with all my heart that my daughters meant well. They just can't understand my pain, because they haven't stood in my shoes, as the saying goes. Not yet!

The other thing for me to change, besides my way of expecting others to rescue me, was to move out of my grandparent's home, and into something more affordable and less demanding. I found myself holding on to an enormous amount of memories of those loved ones, who had long ago passed away. For example, crazy stuff like, hats, coats, many old pocket books, pots and pans, old paintings, and a ton of STUFF! Which simply adds up to, plan old clutter. I was drowning in it unable to separate myself from the past. I doomed myself, of growing and making any real advances in my own life, strangled in the past memories trying to hold on.

You see once my grandparent's passed on, I moved into their home for preservation. Not for myself but for the family's property. To me this home was beautiful, comfortable to say the lease. But the house needed a ton of work, more work than I could afford, now that I am disabled. I wasn't able to maintain, now that I am unable to work which, caused some major anxiety and depression to the point of constant headaches. My primary doctor wanted me to take anti-depressants, but I would not believe I was so depressed to the point of needing medication on a regular basis. I wasn't crazy just stressed out, to the point of it being unhealthy for me physically. Stress is dangerous!

I would always refuse to take any anti-depressants the doctor offered me, from her medicine cabinet. I was always strong and reasonably healthy for the most part, therefore I would decline. The idea of depending on a substance that controlled the way I felt was out of the question. I've had enough people trying to control me, meaning my now ex-husband, on what my thoughts and feelings. Being a mother, daughter, girlfriend or wife made it hard to focus on what I felt and believed in for so many years. I felt restricted to make a move without thinking of others first, and when I did oh man, someone all ways got hurt, even me. People make mistakes and I have made some big ones along the way. I realize now that I don't always make the perfect choices. But they were my choices and life is restricting enough! It took me too long I believe, to figure out who I was as a person. In my 20's then 30's and I can remember even before then, being unsure of who was as a person. Not feeling complete until, my 40's and then I was completely comfortable within myself. Learning my likes and dislikes only to have my emotions stifled down with medication, and confused by treatments of menopause, was a serious move for me to take on as a way of life.

Well, until the recurring Breast Cancer and Hysterectomy that is, talking about having a change, of heart. Herbal anti-depressants became my best friend, but only for a few months while I was experiencing "the change" or menopause. The decision to take these pills became mandatory! Arguing with myself that, it was only going to be for a short period, then and then only because I completely stopped functioning. I was faced with needing the medication to help me with my full blown menopause. Losing sleep and becoming more irritable each day, I just couldn't sleep from the heat building up inside of my body, causing sweat to pore from everywhere, making it difficult to dress.

The crying was ridicules, sporadic at times. Extremely embarrassing because no body understood, what the problem was really. Then combing my hair to make a decent style was also out of the question, my hair was always damp and unmanageable with the menopause. Also going downstairs to greet people became difficult, and all of that was if I were able to pull myself out of the bed. Just forget about doing anything else. The emotions were enormous for me with the onset of "menopause". Although I wake some mornings with great aches and pains from my head, to my toes literally giving me the feeling of being three times my age. This is a good one while all of this is going on I was still looking extremely younger than my true age. The entire thing made it difficult to wake up in the best of moods.

So, there are times when I just don't wake up cheerful. When the first thing I feel is pain. Pain in my fingers, knees, shoulders, neck, hip and even my buttocks the muscles overall hurt, but once the day gets going I begin to feel better I am able to have a normal day filled with all the good stuff that remind me that I am blessed to be alive. Anyway, Things are great now. Don't get me wrong I still struggle with money issues, but I don't worry about repairs on a big house made for a family that was too much for me to manage, or a car that I couldn't afford to maintain alone. I wouldn't have believed it possible, but it is possible to be happy, comfortable and content. Struggling to leave the past in order to move into the future was the best thing I've ever done. At least I know now that I can adjust to change.

Now, I can visit the positive people, places, and things as I chose and not feel the negative repercussions attached, that caused me so much stress and grief of the past that threatened my life. I can enjoy speeding some real quality time with my grandchildren, watching them grow. Before I moved out of my grandparent's home the idea of my spending an hour alone with my grandchildren, or the thought of a weekend visit was too much for me to consider.

Until this summer July 9, 2007, was really the best summer ever because, I was able to comfortably spend some real quality time with my nieces and nephew along with my all of my grandchildren, here in my new home. Seeing them laugh and play was all I had ever wanted. I simply couldn't, enjoy them before, because my health and financial issues just wouldn't allow it, which broke my heart because the children grow so fast and not being able to spend time with my grandchildren knowing others were, really upset me immensely. My pride forced me to act as if this, never bother me and I wanted to save face. Today is a new day and I am happy again! I am finally, to a point in my life where, I am able to join in on some of the fun with the children in our family, contributing again to making new memories for all of us to treasure. A little is way better than nothing. You know, I still have days when I feel slower than normal because of my health, and I can deal with that but to be able to have the children come over and stay for a few days is a wonderful blessing, bringing so much joy.

I have some incredible experiences to remember. Not all bad either, but you know when I am looking back into my life using my journals. I am reliving some frustrating times, feelings and emotions of bad memories, in my battle with cancer. I used them as a way of venting out daily frustration, when I had nobody to really understand. So, I just want remind you that it was not all bad. There were a lot of good times. Easter dinner with everyone together, when I pulled myself together enough to help make the family a simple dinner knowing in my heart that, I should have been resting. Keeping up traditions was very important. My mother and grandmother would have had no problem making this happen for everyone. So, as long as there was a team, Easter super was a success.

I always remember the feeling, when I was pregnant, expecting with both of my daughters. Now that I am older, being a witness to the blessings of giving birth is even more a beautiful than ever. For me the blessing is in being able to be right there in the delivery room watching the birth of the babies in family. God couldn't have smiled on me more than at that very moment, then to have my prayers answered, seeing my own youngest daughter in childbirth and cutting the umbilical cord of her first born, when she's always argued, saying she would never have children reminds me of all the real goodness in the world. I look forward to all the new babies, being born.

To complete a book when I've been reading books written by others all my life, pulling the tooth of my first grandson, by my oldest daughter's child (as my own mother would have had no problem doing). I would run my daughters over to my mother's house so she could pull their teeth, because at the time I just couldn't stand to think of doing it myself.

Today kicking back having a meal and watching movies all day with my little ones means everything to me. Watching them grow up and seeing the great job their mother's are doing with them, takes my breath away. Being blessed to see them use their mothering skills warms my heart and soul. Traveling again, working on a piece of art, taking long walks everyday, getting in on a nice Yoga or Tai Chi class, spending the afternoon walking the neighbors dogs, or spending the day in the neighborhood YMCA, working out in the heated pool and going fishing with my closest friend is, my definition of what 'smelling the roses of life' is all about. A great day for me starts off with that early morning breakfast, and because I am a television junky, I love to watch Good Morning America, Regis & Kelly, then I would go out for a little walk during Rachael Ray, but return to catch The View with Whoopi and then back out to help with the neighbor's dogs until Ellen and then Oprah. Unless I'm up and out early and in the car then I'll listen to Wake up with Whoopi! If I can get some exercise and my favorite shows I am happy, and that is just the early portion of the day.

The evening shows differ from day to day.

If you're ever at a point in your life where you are dwelling hard on holding on and letting go, take a chance, on change. Easing into a new way of life while letting go of the old life, slowly if you need to, was very difficult but rewarding. Use the internet or a cancer support group to find someone in the same situation as you are to make steps in finding a friend to relate and even reach out too. Even further you may find someone you can share a nice condo or apartment. Have someone rent your old place if you're not that comfortable with you decision to make changes. While you seek a place that offers you peace of mind while you are learning to live life on your own terms, in order to find your way. You can get a place just for you if you are single or something for you and that special person in your life. A fresh start over, was what I needed. Don't be afraid to downsize everything! Simplify your life! I believe it is the key. If you aren't happy you can always go back! At least try it . . . Sit down and close your eyes and open up yourself to what, really is stressing you in your life. But let go of that stress! You're life is more important than a stressful job with a bunch of responsibilities.

I was sitting outside on my front porch of my grandparent's house, looking at the grass growing tall, getting out of control and needing to be cut and seeing the two park size tree branches, scraping the roof of the house in the front yard and the other in the back of the house leaning over the wires that crossed over the driveway from house to house. Those branches need to be cut back forced me to realize the greatness of responsibilities hanging on my shoulders. Everything was out of control and it was about to be cold again. Knowing I had no extra money and needed to once again, call on my good friends. Who are busy with their own lives, for more help was too much to expect. Seeing my seventy-two year old lady friend and church mom, cut the grass in my fenced in yard, while I sat watching her from the step, was the final straw. She was healthy enough, since she was healthier than most and willing, I didn't turn down the offer, but I felt uncomfortable all the same. I just didn't want to continue, depending on them for on going help, especially on a house that was never ever going to be mine. I know that my cardiologist gave me strict instructions. Using gardening equipment such as the weed wacker to cut the grass was one of those things, I should not do myself! Deciding that I had no other choice, I would from time to time do it myself and suffer afterwards. Staying in my bed praying the pain away, hard headed and as stubborn as I am, it was time to make some overdue changes. When I would take on cutting the grass myself, I suffered with pain in my arms, you'll never imagine. Only God knows why I never ended up with swelling of in my arms. I just could not want to ask for the help anymore, and I needed to keep the lawn up like all the other home owners on the block.

I owed it to my self to move on, into a different and new life after all that I've been through. Considering letting go of some extremely sentimental, and personal things that belonged to my dear mother, grandparent's and even my youngest aunt, was very hard but worth it because it allowed me a chance to shed some superficial stress, and possibly a year or two to my life. Deciding to keep a few choice pieces of their lives instead of holding on to everything was not easy for me. Learning to alter my own life in order to smell the roses, smile and laugh again caused some grief in the beginning, but the end result was again worth it. Finding my way to have some harmless fun again has turned out to be my greatest decision ever!

It's now December, 2007, Christmas one week away and again my heart is heavy, knowing almost everyone is aggressive about this affliction that taunts my family and needed to be tested for the mutation gene has been, except for a few who most likely are afraid. Still, testing is needed for their children's sake. There was only one person other than my self showing to have the mutation BRCA1 gene, and that person is my twenty-nine year old daughter. My first born has the gene and she has recently discovered a lump in her breast, after close examination by her physician, she was informed that there were two lumps. That lump tested positive for cancer. I accompanied my daughter for the consultation concerning the various test required before the surgery and treatment plan. I watch my daughter as she sits in a bit of shock, every now and then asking a question or smiling when I made an attempt to lighten the moment. Every now and then I can see her slip off into that dark world deep inside herself. A world I know very well. I'm sure my daughter did not know what to ask, as the doctor asked if there were any questions. There is a ton of information to receive all at once, much more a patient can take at one time. It all sounds like gibber after a while. I feel blessed to be able to ask or answer any questions, the doctor or my daughter would need to know. At one point she worried over the fact that she may have passed the gene over to her daughter. Tears filled both of us when I sat there knowing I was the reason she was stricken with this illness. I also worried over the possibility thinking that I may have passed the gene, to not only my granddaughter but to my grandsons as well. The last thing I want to think of is the next generation having this gene. We forget that breast cancer not only affects the females, it can and does affect the males, and if the males test positive for the mutation gene they risk the chance of having any type of cancer. It breaks my heart to know that I've passed this gene on to my oldest daughter and I pray not to any of my grandchildren. I've always wished that my mother, grandmother or aunt was here to walk me through my battles, and God has allowed me to be a blessing in my daughter's life by being here for her in her battle. I pray to my father God above to please strip this gene away from my entire family and please watch over my daughter, drape her with the armor she will need to stay strong in her battles concerning this affliction. Amen.

Dedications to Marnita Kidd

"I am sorry you have been going through this thing called "Cancer", I believe that some races, are ran fast and some are ran very slow, the race for you has been very slow but remember that each day that you are still here, is a day that God has made for you. Your body is missing out on a beautiful spirit, if your body can understand that you have been fighting to take care of it, nurturing, loving it, and being at peace with it.

Marnita you have been so strong in spirit, this is what we will all remember the most.

Let this Valentine's Day be about the spirit in your heart . . ."

Always in the spirit,

Juanita

A letter from Tyra

I was very young when I met Marnita. It was around 1993, I was hanging out with family and friends. Marnita came across as a very loving quiet woman. As time passed with different outings, I discovered that Marnita wasn't as quiet as I thought and we became close friends. We talked everyday about anything and everything. Marnita told me, she lived through my life listening to my life stories. I loved telling her stories never holding back on any details. I remember a ski trip Marnita, her oldest daughter and my self attended together. The tree of us shared a room at the resort. We had fun living on the wild side. It was the funniest trip. But the highlight for me was when Marnita all dressed up in her winter jacket, struggled to climb the hill with her snow tube. She got about ¾ the way up the hill when all of a sudden all you can hear is "Oh no my tube!" Marnita was standing there watching her tube slide all the way back down the hill. A nice man ran after her tube to bring it back to her. It was funny to see. This trip brought us even closer as friends, each time I watch the tape of that ski trip I laugh so hard. I consider Marnita my confidant. She always listened to me without judgment. I was one of Marnita's friends who stayed beside her with the loss of her mother, while she was grieving. One night I spent the night with her following the funeral of her mother, it was rough for me as well, but my main objective was to be there for her. When I was told about Marnita's illness, I was taken back. I was very concerned and didn't know how to cope with talking to her about it. Her knowing me very well, she took control of the conversation making it easy on me. She filled me in on every detail of her illness. I talked to her daily, as a friend for support, telling her I loved her. Even after she told me about her illness she still wanted to talk to me about my problems as she was a very strong individual. I visited Marnita the day before she went to have surgery. I still have the picture, I will never forget day. A couple of years later, Marnita tell me she's sick again, we reacted the same way as before but this time, because we were prepared. I could see that Marnita was very upset that she had to go through this all over again. But she had support from many other friends and family. Here it is 2006 and Marnita tells me cancer has returned for the third time and she's concerned that it may have spread. Her doctors tell her of the numerous procedures to help her. To me it takes a hell of a strong woman to have all of these things done. I must admit I didn't understand fully but after talking with others concerning her treatment plans, health issues and recovery, I got how strong she really was. Marnita had at least five different surgeries this year alone, with some support beside her. We don't talk as much as we used to but we have a friendship like no other, which is unconditional love and friendship for one another.

Tyra

Learning to separate my self from the world by turning off the telephone, not answering the door and shutting off the internet without guilt, helped me to focus on the importance of life, and that's me!

Marnita Ellen Kidd breast cancer survivor since 1998 and still fighting . . .

There are very few people that I have met in this world that get "Life" the understanding of its purpose and how to live each day with thanks and gratitude. Very few people have yet to learn how to enjoy life, honor life, and love life. This is the best way I can describe Marnita.

Marnita has been my friend and spiritual sister for many years, we met in 1995, over the years we have had the opportunity to share our experience's and thoughts on what life means to us, sure there were many storms on sunny days and no gas money when the car needed to run, but in light of that, it was still a part of life.

I have no doubt that Marnita's life story will give someone the courage to live in the moment of "Life". Marnita continues to be a light that shines on the darkest of days.

Lyrics of a song . . . .

"I am not my clothes, I am not my hair, and I am not this skin"

I am the spirit that lives within

                                                                              Juanita

A letter from my good friend Kelly . . .

Marnita, What a great opportunity to tell you what you mean to me!

Here it goes:

I met Marnita through my sister, who she was friends with first. I knew right away that she was something special and I wanted her to be my friend too. In this mixed up, crazy world, you don't often come across people of Marnita's quality. I saw that quality in her and decided we should be friends. You know how they say that little children can see right through adults and see whether a person is truly good? Well, when my daughter and Marnita spent some time with us here in New Hampshire and McKenzie got so attached to her, right away! I can still see McKenzie cuddling up to her on the sofa, and I can still see the joy on McKenzie's face, joy just to be sitting near "her" new friend. She called Marnita "little girl", because McKenzie could see right through Marnita and saw kindness, gentleness and a purity that you only find in "little girls". I admire Marnita because she has had such a tough go of it with her health, but she rarely complains and she is fighting the good fight so we her family and friends are not robbed of her beauty love and intelligence!

Kelly

My good friend Dwayne wrote:

Dwayne says:

When life is kicking me in the butt and I think I can't go on any more. I stop and think about Marnita. If anyone should feel like they can't go on any longer she should. But she doesn't. With all the bad breaks life has given her she continues to have a positive outlook on life.

So when I hear people talk about how bad they have it, or how rotten life has been to them. I just shake my head and think of Marnita and say to myself, "If you only knew how good you have it". Marnita really keeps me from feeling sorry for my self.

Because she can keep going, I can too!

Dwayne

Sheila's letter read . . .

Hello Marnita,

Marnita you are sister/girl to me. You are like my sister who I can share anything with, without you judging me, and you are my girl, because you have always had my back. I admire you so much as you dealt with your cancer experiences. You have been so strong and kept a positive attitude through your experiences, and steal had time to support your family, friends and be there for us. I live you so much, thank you for always being there for me, supporting me and never judging me

You are the best.

Love always Sheila

THE ROSE

It's soft to the touch,
So delicate and sweet
To the love is much,
Who receives this treat
Its natural beauty is amazing to behold,
Thoughts of purity render the soul
It thirsts with delight,
Striking to see at first sight
Be careful when you reach,
Although it's as velvet as a peach
The slenderness of her stretch,
Is known to pierce the flesh
The fragrance will fill your soul,
With the many colors to behold
The shades can clearly attest,
To the emotions your hearts desires to express

I've learned a few life lessons from a couple of very close friends in my life. Considering the fact that they were older and wiser or we shared similar life experiences. I am happy I was smart enough to accept and appreciate what they were teaching me, when I needed to learn, which has helped me get through life thus far. My most adored girlfriend is Cherry. We became telephone girlfriends when she moved away. She's offered me the greatest emotional support being a strong willed her self. From the beginning of our friendship, she would often console me from a nurse point of view on my health, when we were fighting breast cancer at the same times. We took that walk together in the fight for life, and more than once. She understood exactly what I felt in every way, winning a few battles with caner herself, and having that nurse's view point on things turned out to be very helpful.

She would verbally argue with me in order to convince me that she understood what I wanted so desperately to tell her as I was explaining out of sheer frustration. I was finding it difficult from all the different emotions filling up in my body, concerning family, friend's, neighbors, on top of the actual battles with cancer and even life to cope. She has her own way of making me feel, that it was all normal, especially when I was so upset and I believed I couldn't get my point across to anyone else concerning the things I was feeling or experiencing. I was extremely emotional, frightened and she understood everything! It makes a big difference to know someone understands, even if it is one person . . .

My first letter about my good friend Cherry on 07-26-2007 reads:

"It turns out that Cherry's sprained ankle was far more than we could expect. She has been diagnosed with cancer metastases throughout her body (brain, lung, liver, bone—and probably elsewhere). She is currently at Dove House 292 Stoner Avenue Westminster, MD 21157 which is an inpatient hospice center. She is much more comfortable now that we are out of the hospital and the staff and the facility are extremely nice. She's got her country music playing all the time and has been able to take care of a lot of business that she felt needed done, vs. a vs. the family. She went into the hospital last Friday and her family was down from Philly for the weekend and several are returning this weekend. She is very much at peace with what is happening with her and is looking forward to a better place with no pain. Call the hospice, but I don't have the phone number on me right now. I don't always answer, in part because the reception is sporadic and it sometimes just tells me I've missed calls instead of ringing, but I have it at all times and will return your call as soon as convenient."

My heart drops in disbelief.

The second letter read:

"Cherry passed away at about 10:30 pm Thursday night 08-09-07. She was peaceful and comfortable and is no doubt enjoying a rest that she deserves. Thank you for your thoughts and prayers during this time."

A note to my girlfriend Cherry who lost her battle to cancer: Rest in peace I know I will see you again . . .

Cancer is not prejudice, it doesn't care what you have been through in your life nor where you plan on going in your future, are we all one family when it comes down to these afflictions.

We say a cat's has nine lives. I've heard someone say "she's only been dyeing for years", referring to my own existence. Disregarding and not understanding how difficult it is for me to get from one day to the next. I Thanks God I am blessed to say I am still here, although I have really bad days and other challenges with my health. It's still a blessing to be alive!

Blessings come in the most unforgettable ways, bringing special friendships with others, offering help when I was in great need.

God sends you angels when you need them and then he can take them away once their job is done

Embracing where I am in life today comes hard but well worth the fight. Often comes with doubt, and contradicting emotions concerning the battle.

I know that there are people who have had other types of challenges concerning their health. I simply wanted to share some of my experiences, hoping that I can make a difference in someone else's life. This will make the experience I had with my afflictions worth going through. If I can help one person to realize that they can endure and survive any thing with strong faith, in order to enjoy life again, then my job is done. This Christmas 2006 is very special to me. I knew seeing the way this year started off, this year was going to be a challenge, not just for me but for everyone. I continued to say "this was going to be my year", and it has been my year. I was forced to spend this year focused on myself. Learning Tai Chi, Yoga and exercising on a regular basis taught me how to tap into the simple positive things in my life, and to shake off the negative unhealthy things that cause an illness like cancer to take over and feed on the stress that I know I hold inside of me.

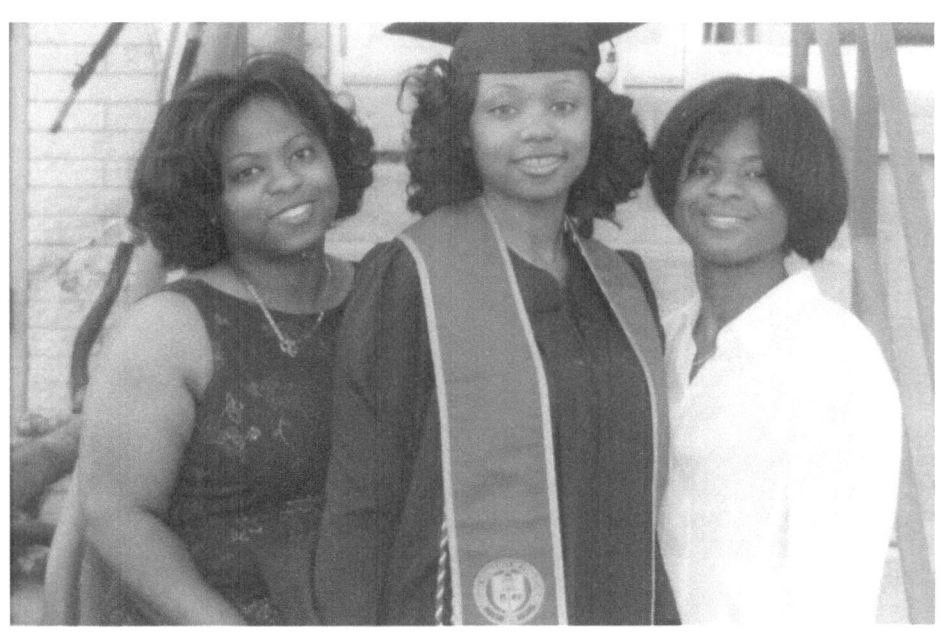

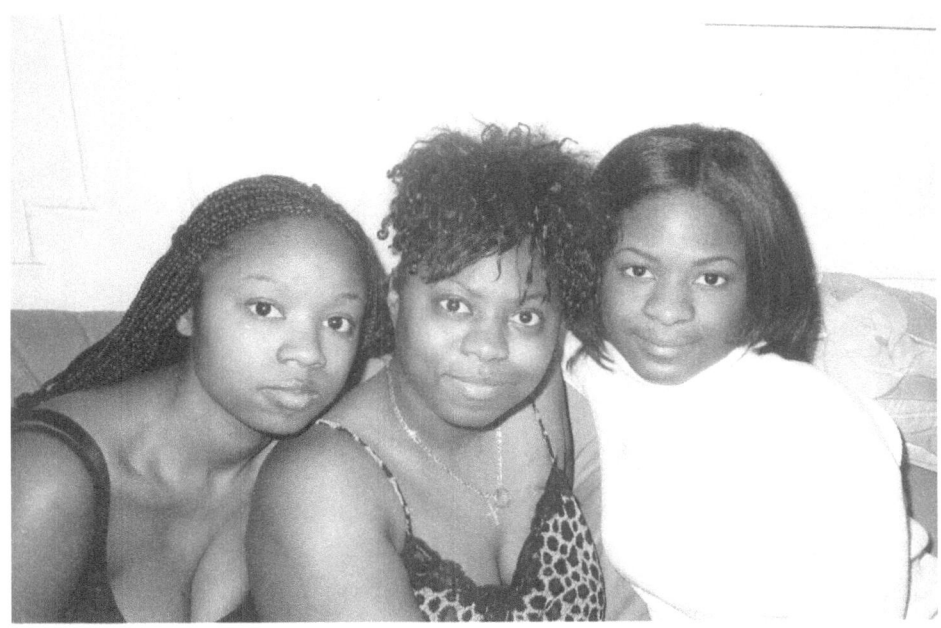

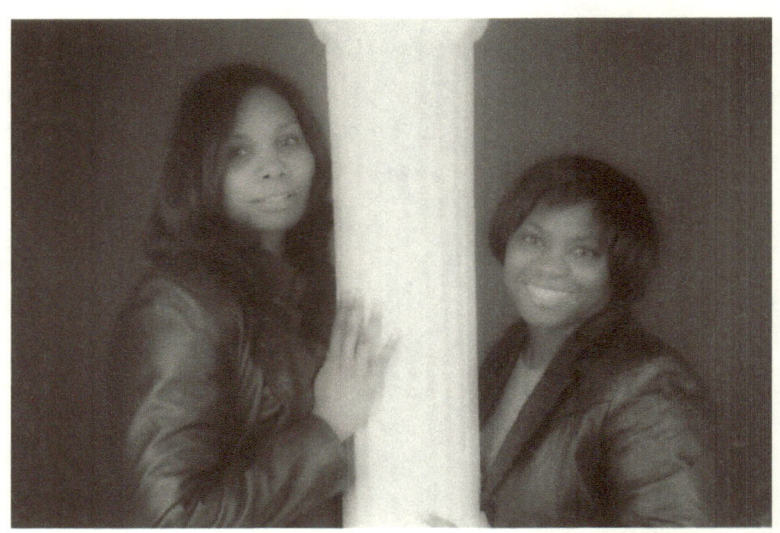

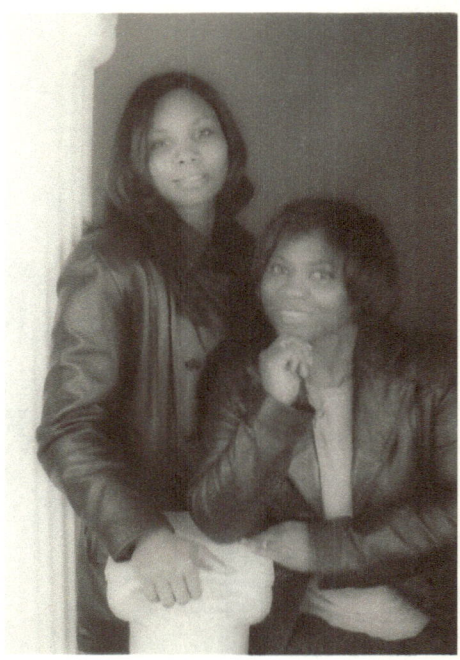

Extended blessings—The gift of friendship with others offering help when I was in need.

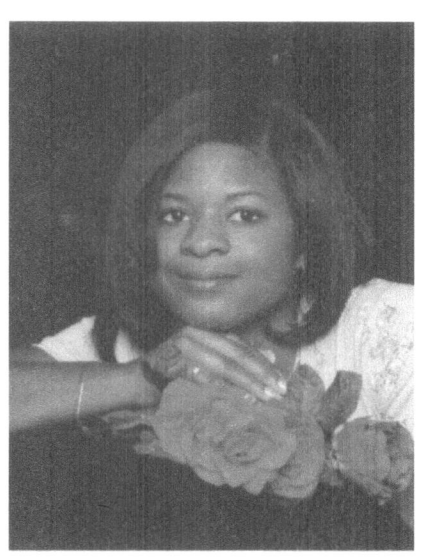

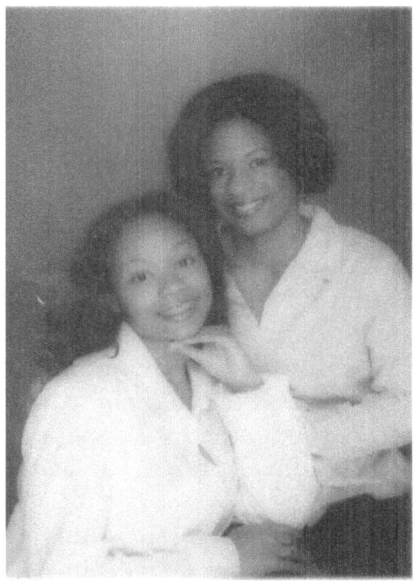

My Beautiful Daughters
(Right) Tyesha Love
(Left) Candice Love

I Love You Always . . . .

Mom

This Christmas I watched people running around picking out their Christmas trees, decorating their homes, shopping for food and gifts to go under the tree, with their Christmas music filling the air. Everyone's pretty much competing with one another to be the best decorated home or to give the most expensive gifts. Preparing for the traditional celebration of this holiday, but it's different for me. I on the other hand enjoy seeing people preparing for Christmas but I'm not in the traditional mood for this day. I feel extremely humbled just being alive. This year I find myself submerged into the spiritual meaning of Christmas.

My only real Christmas wish this year is to have everyone surrounding me on Christmas day, spending time together. I would like everyone to grab pillows and take a seat on the floor, to humble ourselves as one, in order to remember our blessings.

This Christmas is extremely special to me because I am here to see it. This time last year I was concerned about a third lump that appeared in my breast. There was a few times where I thought, making it through this year just wasn't possible. Being so close to seeing this year end makes my fight with cancer official. I've won! I'm still here to look into the faces of those I love with all my heart. I'm not perfect but God is good to me. He has stripped me of my outer self to give me eyes to see and appreciate what, being here is supposed to mean.

The best gift to me is from my father above. He has given me the gift, of allowing me to see so many things this year, things I would have missed out on. I've been given a deeper spiritual growth, in dealing with the fears of my health issues, and a blessing to witness the birth of another grandchild.

God has blessed me to have a clearer understanding in the meaning of, the strength in prayer, undying faith, unconditional love, growth, the importance of forgiveness, to embrace change, endure loneliness, life and death, sharing, selfishness, greed, pain and to endure suffering. I was blessed to see the old go and the new come in, and to be able to feel what real support, acceptance, empathy, sympathy, friendship, and what real togetherness really feels like. Also to see what unconditional really means.

I've learned many things this year alone. A single year can hold a lot of things that tend to feel more negative than positive. Learn to ride the wave of the negative things, but do not holding on to them for longer than you need. Being humble in the lessons of life is half the battle. These things are going to happen just experience them and let them go . . . . Don't try to waste time trying to figure out the "Why's" or "how's" of things. Accept and move on, quick. The blessing is to be able to believe in something enough to over come, and know that you can survive, with faith. When something doesn't work out the way you plan, force the issue or look down in defeat, it doesn't mean any thing negative, when you do not get what you wanted. It just means that, it wasn't meant to be, simple as that. It also means that there is a different blessing in the making that is especially for you. Unanswered prayers are blessings too. Remember that!

I know that it's tradition to have a Christmas tree, the sent of pine in the air, gifts under the tree, Christmas lights twinkling, home cooked food and other decorations all around. A house full of friends and family. This year is very special for me, that I only wish to spend it in a very simply and humble way. To appreciate the true blessings this Christmas. The true blessing this year for me is . . . The gift of life . . . .

I thank God for allowing me to be here another year.

It's Feb. 2007 and a few days ago I was blessed to find another lump in between new breast, just under my chest bone. I've already called and have been seen by my oncology surgeon and the CT Scans have already started . . . . Please don't be afraid to make that first telephone call as soon as you can it may save your life . . . . Catching cancer early makes a big difference. For me the fight goes on . . . .

This year has shown to be a very special year, for many reasons. Special doesn't have to mean perfect nor easy. Which, we all know nothing in life is perfect and nor easy. Easy is something this year hasn't been. I don't know anyone who has survived breast cancer three times besides my self, let alone four times if you consider cancer cells in her uterus, on top of that while dealing with congestive heart failure, encountering one surgery after another. Please realize if you haven't already, if you really want anything in life, "it's not going to be easy", an old saying but very true.

I retired as a Bursar from Temple University now on Social Security Disability. Feeling even more restricted than ever financially, I work out ways to get through the days. I can still exercise and fill my days going to the YMCA, which offers financial assistant for those who qualify. I'm not afraid to use generic brand medicine to stretch my once a month income.

Fighting for life over death once again, which was difficult for so many reasons but still worth the fight. Some of us just have to work harder at staying alive, and making more of an effort to make the most out of life. Where others take life for granted, easing their way through without the true awareness, of all the simple beauty and blessings surrounding them. I had to almost lose my life three times, in order to wake up and see what life and love was. I mean love on a deeper level. The love of innocence like in a baby or a child, and in nature like the many different types of trees and plants, the smell of fresh air, the ducks, dears, rabbits, or stray animals. It's very important for me to enjoy everything in my life.

I was reading The New York Times on Sunday, August 26th 2007, while sitting outside waiting a table at an indoor, outdoor restaurant. The article spoke of famous people in midlife, wrestling with issues of personal worth. These people shared their life list and goals. This article was about making your own personal list of things. Things you would like to do before you die. Harsh but real, and I could appreciate the article. Again, I know this is hard to imagine but necessary all the same. I learned two things that day from this article. One was that I needed to make out my own life list and that "We tend to feel happy when we make progress towards our goals and anxious when we don't." Which justify my anxiety with writing this book, making it easier to continue and not give up, when I didn't feel this project was going as well as it should. This article shares that "List like these shows a universal longing for adventure, fulfillment and grace." So, it is normal for me to feel anxiety when I am pressed to complete something that is really only important to me. So, don't give up or into the challenges of your own list. Make sure you stop to make out your life list and check them off periodically. When you pitch the path through life that's more for filling to you, ask yourself this question. What **is** life supposed to be like for you?

I had to put together my own life list. It's simple nothing too complicate to accomplish. I would like to share my list with you now.

My life list which is not in order consists of the following along with few other personal one's that are not mentioned.

1. I would like to own a little convertible.
2. I would like to complete a nice art painting.
3. I would like to fly first class to Paris France.
4. I would like to visit Canada.
5. I would like to own a bed and breakfast.
6. I would like to learn Spanish.
7. I would like to learn to play the guitar.
8. I would like to learn to ride a motorcycle.
9. I would like to go Ice skating.
10. I would like to take a dance class.
11. I would like to be my goal weight of 130 lbs.
12. I would like to make frequent trips to any Island, even by way of a cruise.
13. I would like to be consistent and exercise three to four times every week.
14. I would like to complete my own book and have it published.
15. I would like to be confident in my practice with Yoga and Tai Chi once a day on my own.
16. I would like to update my passport.
17. Not having full coverage health benefits after retiring from Temple University, restricting me from the luxury of dental care. I would like to go to an orthodontist or dentist. There is nothing like having a

tooth ache while you are going through your healing treatment in your battle. I had the experience of having extreme pain during my healing process. Needing some bridge work and not being able to afford the price of an orthodontist. Twice this happened to me in 2006 and with no insurance to cover a dentist I made my way down Broad Street in Philadelphia. In the dark, on both of those early morning trips, to Temple Dental School. Standing on the stairs, in the dark and in the cold at 6:00 a.m. with others in pain, I took my chances on being robbed or attacked going there alone. A bad tooth ache will make you weigh out the fear of someone robbing you. I would have done anything to get those teeth out! I was extremely desperate, praying that I wouldn't get turned away for that day's count of accepted patients. I hid my cash needed for the extraction and watched my back. My only request was to have the teeth pulled out! I had enough pain to last me the rest of that year, and a tooth ache wasn't in the plan. By the afternoon I was free of a few of teeth, I wished at one time I was able to keep, but happy.

Not having medical insurance has taken me through many other changes. Working as a Medical Assistant in a small clinic, I've seen first hand the different treatment a person receives just because they have one type of insurance or another. I only have one insurance so, walking in to the front desk to register receiving the question of my I have your insurance cards and only handing in one, takes me to a new level of care. This is when you get full treatment because I have Medicare as a primary, but no secondary, which is fine for the 80%, but for the 20% balance that is my responsibility, isn't good. Knowing that I will be stuck with this balance bill that I already know I can't afford makes me question taking test I know I need, fearing that 20% bill. But I walk in to the doctor's office now with the attitude of a person holding a primary and secondary insurance, because I don't care! I need the test or care of the specialist so I go in anyway with the idea that I will pay what I can, when I can, because it's my life and I need and deserve to have the same care as a person with full coverage. It's not my fault that, I am no longer working! It is not my fault that I don't have full coverage insurance! It is not my fault that I am not healthy! But it is my job to demand quality care for my life's existence. My English is not what it should be and I know this, wondering if this project was a good idea was a constant worry. Frustration set in, when there was no computer to work, knowing I didn't even own my own computer. Anxiety pushed me down when the publishing company made demands for their money and I really did not have it! I would have been very upset with myself if I didn't complete this project.

You may think this is crazy, but I would receive different signs from people who didn't know me offering encouragements, and fortune cookies that read "Reach for your dreams", "Don't be surprised by the emergence of undiscovered talents"; "Luck happens when hard work meets opportunity." "Bide your time, for success is near", "The secret of vast riches begins with a single penny." "Your example will inspire others." And "There is beauty in simplicity." It was crazy but every fortune cookie had a real message inside of it that was just for me, when I was in great doubt, ready to toss my book project into the trash. Considering that it's now October, 2007 breast cancer month adds even more pressure but more encouragement. I'm greatly encouraged to complete this venture. So, for better or worse I can now cross this project, off of my life list and move on to next thing.

I've always wanted to volunteer my services, you know contribute something? I just never seem to have enough money in order to make a donation. Whenever I receive one of those forms in the mail from The Beast Cancer Foundations, or their Fund Raisers Committees", I'm filled with guilt. I want to do something but wasn't able to financially. I never really was able to give money, but knowing first hand about the benefits attached to this donation, I wanted to give back and offer something to others in their fight as a way of support. One day I received a telephone call from The Linda Creed Breast Cancer Foundation, with a special request.

It was explained to me that they were running a fund raiser and needed a few people to come downtown to tell their own stories, on surviving breast cancer. I was honored and nervous at the same time, but having the idea that there were going to be others speaking on stage, I soon got over my anxiety. Because if they could stand up and tell their stories so could I. Remember the day so clear. I wore a nice tea length black dress, with a beautiful shawl that was my mothers. I figured, this was a special invitation and I believe my mother would have been proud of me to follow through. I had my best wig, covering my baldness offering me some security and confidence, while masking how exposed and vulnerable, I really felt inside.

If course I arrived early as I always do, to find only a few people from the organization. They were busy, still setting up getting ready for the event. I explained to them who I was and they made me feel very comfortable. I sat there reading over my speech waiting for the other speakers. Until it was made clear that, I was the only guest speaker for their fundraiser. People started coming in and taking seats. I started to sweat under my wig. I never felt comfortable reading, in front of a bunch of people or anything like or close to public speaking. How was I going to pull this one off? I really wanted to run out of the door! Being the trooper that I was, holding my not so well written speech in my lap, trying to look confident, I re-read over my papers. Whishing I had not written so much. My heart jumped out of my chest, when they called my name out, to come up on stage. Everyone started clapping, and smiling. All I could this of was "Oh my goodness!" If I could have turned into someone else at that very moment I would have!

I remember telling myself to breathe once on stage in front of the podium and that's what I did. Every single chance there was, more often than needed, I took a breath! A long slow breath to calm myself down, with those obvious breaks in between my sentences. I didn't want to rush my speech seeing, that I put so much energy into it, and there wasn't any one else to leave time for anyway. So, I stood there behind the podium, with papers in hand wanting to faint. If you can imagine it, all eyes on me, as I talked about my story, my experiences with breast cancer. Their face swelled with tears, men and women, cried and laughed, shaking their heads while, reminiscing from their own experiences. It was hard for me to contain my own tears seeing them react to my little speech. Mostly because it was painful to relive out loud in front of a room filled with people I never met before and the story was true concerning the experiences I had with breast cancer. I made it through the speech, rushing the end a little more deciding I was ready for the attention on me to be over and all of a sudden, people stepped on to the stage wanting to hug and kiss me, almost knocking my wig off of my head. I had to hold the wig on to my head! We were all crying, smiling, and embracing one another. It was truly a great experience! And at the end of the ceremony, I was presented with an in scripted crystal bowl "L.C.B.C.F. 2002 Honoree". Although I had no family members there to witness this special day with me, I was very proud of myself.

You know what? I know my mother would have been proud.

I don't look at having this gene as a punishment. I believe God has his way of making us stop and take notice to the simple things in life. It's just his way of saying I need you to take a look and really see all of the forgotten goodness. He would not punish or curse us in this way. He loves all of us and my battles were a universal example of Gods lessons, leaving me to be rich in soul and spirit. I know that I am a witness to what God can do . . . .

A HUG

You can do it here and there,
People do it everywhere
You do it at the door,
And even on the floor
You can get one on the run
And they're really so much fun
They're really nice at night
When you're holding someone real tight
You can often sneak a kiss
When you really feel missed
You can do this to everyone
Or to that very special one
Children tend to grown up and miss
On holidays you see a lot of this
Wonderful to share
When a persons in despair
When it lifts your spirits like a rocket
You'll wish you could place it in your pocket
If it's real you'll know it from the start
Keeping it close to your heart

Acknowledgments

I would like to make sure I say thanks, to the caregivers and friends in my life, who sat with me making sure I knew I was loved and not alone. I recognize the sacrifices, made in order to be there for someone struggling with health issues. I know it is a difficult position to be in, especially on a daily basis. Thanks for enduring along with me, in my times of fear, doubt, confusion, anxiety, pain, and venerability. I also want to say thanks for standing by me, with my overwhelming emotions of insecurity, abandonment and feelings of uselessness. I know on occasions that I have lashed out towards those closest to me, while I was in my battles with cancer, not knowing what to expect next. Please know that I love you, and I am really grateful and blessed to have you all, in my life.

Thank you to those who extended themselves using emails or telephone calls to stay in touch, because we live so far away from each other. No matter, I just wanted to say thanks to you for hanging in there with me, all the way through. Your act of selflessness and constant encouragement meant everything to me and I greatly appreciate every thing. I don't know what I would have done without your help and support. Thank you for giving me a positive, atmosphere of support, offering me the healthiest, successful, recovery necessary. Many blessings to you always . . . .

I was strongly inspired to write this book by my close friend, her relentless spirituality encouraged me to challenge my fears to become "a writer and author", as an attempt to share my story with the world. Many thanks to you always, my sister in spirit, Mrs. Juanita Johnson . . .

Ms. Sharrie A. Wilson, Thank you for supporting my dreams. And sharing your life with me making use of your automobiles, knowing I couldn't afford to keep up with my used broken down. You have taken the pressure and smothering responsibilities off of me, when I was trying to further stretch money, I really didn't have in order to maintain them. Thanks for building a door into the basement, to bring in the beautiful new washer and dryer you purchased, to save me from hauling laundry back and forth to get them cleaned, when it was too hot or too cold outside. Thanks for trying hard to make my grandparents home comfortable, making the floors shine like water, when it was finically useless. Thanks for treating my family and friends to my wonderful, surprise birthday gathering. The dinner at Sotto Varalli's Restaurant, in downtown Philadelphia, was a great choice, creating unforgettable memories, a gift to cherish for a life time.

Most of all thanks including me in your move to West Chester, Pennsylvania, offering me a new home and a breath of fresh air, that fills my life with hopes of nothing but positive things to come. When I felt my life was at an end, you've opened up a world of stress free living and piece of mind, giving me a new beginning, a new start. Many, many blessings to you always for all that you have done and still do . . . Blessings to you also . . .

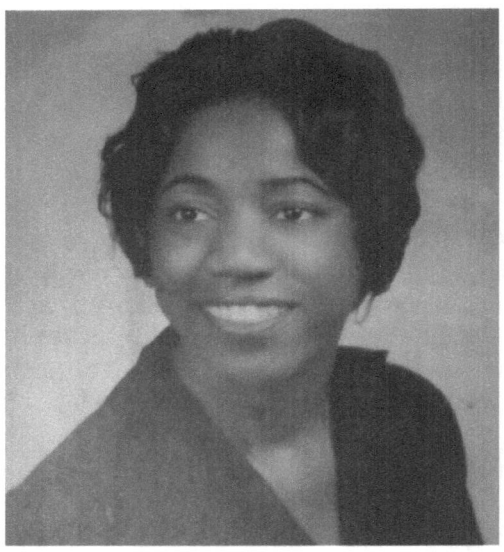

Mrs. Joyce Kidd